UGLY FOOD

TIM WHARTON AND RICHARD HORSEY

UGLY FOOD

Overlooked and Undercooked

HURST & COMPANY, LONDON

First published in the United Kingdom in 2016 by
C. Hurst & Co. (Publishers) Ltd.,
41 Great Russell Street, London, WC1B 3PL

Printed in the United Kingdom by Bell & Bain Ltd, Glasgow

Distributed in the United States, Canada and Latin America by
Oxford University Press, 198 Madison Avenue, New York, NY 10016,
United States of America.

A Cataloguing-in-Publication data record for this book
is available from the British Library.

9781849046862 hardback

This book is printed using paper from registered sustainable
and managed sources.

www.hurstpublishers.com

p. 18 Lyrics from 'Octopus I love you' by Dalmatian Rex and the Eigentones reproduced
with permission.

CONTENTS

RECITES

GIBLETS

CONVERSION TABLES

DRY		LIQUID	
Metric	Imperial	Metric	Imperial
8g	1/4oz	1 tsp/5ml	1/6fl oz
15g	1/2oz	1 tbsp/15ml	1/2fl oz
30g	1oz	30ml	1fl oz
60g	2oz	60ml	2fl oz
90g	3oz	90ml	3fl oz
120g	4oz	120ml	4fl oz
150g	5oz	150ml	5fl oz
180g	6oz	300ml	10fl oz
210g	7oz	450ml	15fl oz
240g	8oz	560ml	1 pint/20fl oz
1kg	2lb 1oz	750ml	25fl oz
1.5kg	3lb 2oz	850ml	30fl oz
2kg	4lb 2oz	1 litre	35fl oz

OVEN TEMPERATURES

°C	°F	gas mark
130	275	1
150	300	2
160	325	3
180	350	4
190	375	5
200	400	6
220	425	7
230	450	8
250	475	9

ACKNOWLEDGEMENTS

We've been thinking about this book for several years and the ideas it contains have been evolving for some time. We hope they have ended up the better for it; like, say, traditional balsamic vinegar, which emerges, rich and complex, after 25 years aging in mulberry and juniper casks; or *jamón ibérico de pellota*, cured and dried in airy, cavernous lofts for 36 months to melting, silken perfection; or hunks of putrefying, urea-ridden Greenland shark, buried underground, leeching their ammoniac stench on the way to becoming the Icelandic delicacy *hakárl*. (Well, maybe not too much like rotten shark, to be brutally honest with our Icelandic friends, but this is a book about expanding horizons, after all...).

A number of publishers considered our ideas at various stages during their fermentation, and not all were convinced by our pitch to champion the ugly and overlooked. We'd like to thank Michael Dwyer for agreeing to take the project on, and Alasdair Craig who understood immediately what we were trying to achieve, and who did much to improve the quality of the final brew. Special thanks to Tanya Ghosh for capturing visually the idea that ugly food has its own kind of beauty. We're grateful to Jon de Peyer, Alison Alexanian and Daisy Leitch at Hurst for all their hard work. Finally, we'd like to thank Darra Goldstein, Jill Norman and Gwen Robinson, for being early champions of the book.

Needless to say, none of these people wishes to take responsibility for our jokes, complaints about which should be directed to us.

Tim Wharton and Richard Horsey, 2016

PREFACE

Ugly Food is a cookery book with a difference; not only is it about neglected or despised foods, it also throws light on the influence of science, psychology and history on what we eat. But it is not a treatise; there are light-hearted diversions into poetry, myth, fiction and film to show how some of our Anglo-Saxon superstitions, fears and revulsions about certain foods have arisen.

Supermarket packaging has further distanced us from the origins of our food, but we are now turning away from this and gradually becoming more adventurous – foraging for wild greens and fungi, buying pigs and ox cheeks from the butcher. Mediterranean and Asian restaurants offer dishes of innards, octopus, goose barnacles, pigs trotters. Fergus Henderson's *Nose to Tail Eating* is at the top of the list of 1000 Best Cookbooks – these are all encouraging signs that interest in these flavourful and often inexpensive foods is growing. Many were eaten regularly by our forebears, and they are prized in other parts of the world. The Victorians ate broiled kidneys, fried lambs brains and sweetbreads for breakfast. Octopus has star status in Japan, in Greece, in Provence.

Tim and Richard are passionate home cooks and their enthusiasm for these forgotten or underrated ingredients is infectious. I hope their appetising recipes, drawn from all parts of the world, will tempt you to put these once ignored foods on the table.

Jill Norman, 2016

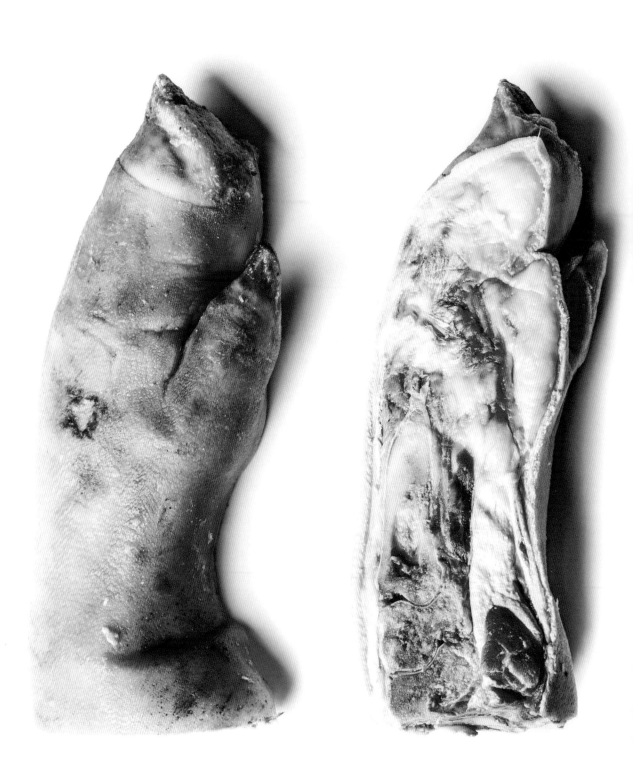

1. INTRODUCTION

Overlooked and undercooked

Octopus is delicious. It's not just good, or nice, or tasty, it's absolutely delicious. Cooked properly, octopus arms have the texture of lobster, perhaps even scallop. They're firm and meaty, but tender. The flavour is hard to describe, and depends a great deal not only on how the octopus has been cooked, but on how it has been prepared before being cooked. Strangely, it doesn't taste remotely like its close cephalopod relation – the squid. It has a subtle, sweet and salty flavour, redolent of the sea.

Arrive late at a fishmonger's shop in the UK and all the pristine-white fillets of vulnerable cod and haddock will be gone. Some of the more expensive 'prime' fish will remain: sole, turbot, sea bass and brill are hardly everyday ingredients. But how many of you notice that nestling deep in the ice, curled up in the back corner of the huge marble slab, are the few octopuses that were landed the night before? And how many of you who notice them consider buying them, and realise they can be cooked and eaten over the next few days in any number of delicious ways?

Of course, we shouldn't complain, but we are at a complete loss as to why, when octopus is half the price of even the cheaper fish, and can provide a sustainable alternative to endangered species, people shy away from this wonderful ingredient. Even the local fishermen view them with a degree of distaste. Octopuses break into lobster and crab pots and are widely regarded as by-catch (that is, the unwanted creatures you end up with in addition to those you're actually trying to catch). A huge increase in the catch in the South of England in the last century was described as a 'plague' of octopus. In the UK, people just don't eat them.

There are many ingredients which, like octopus, are overlooked by Anglo-Saxon cuisines. Rabbits and Squirrels are plentiful – indeed, in many areas they

1

are pests – but despite the fact that they offer tasty, cheap and sustainable alternatives to commercially produced meats, few people eat rabbit and almost no one eats squirrel. Some of the tastiest and most sustainable fish happen to be Ugly Fish: gurnard, garfish, horse mackerel (or scad), catfish, eel-pout and many more. Yet, as with octopus, shoppers are still primarily attracted to those safe, faceless (and often unsustainable) fillets.

And there are many animal parts that consumers are fearful of – worrying that they are difficult to prepare, difficult to cook, or just downright unpalatable. Offal, of course, is one such category, although it is true that offal can be a very demanding ingredient and many people simply don't like the taste of kidneys, liver or tripe, even when prepared well. But other under-appreciated animal parts are a different story. Cheeks and Feet (ox and pig cheeks, cow-heel, pig trotters, chicken feet to name a few) are wonderful: the Boeuf Bourguignon you cook with ox cheeks will be the best you have ever served. Giblets are great too. They are now rarely eaten, but every home cook used to be familiar with them back in the days when birds were bought from the butcher rather than the supermarket (even if they were often used only to add flavour to stuffing or gravy). And there are many overlooked Ugly Veg that make up for in flavour what they lack in outward appearance: celeriac, Hamburg parsley, Jerusalem artichoke, mangel-wurzel and more. Why shoppers are more attracted to expensive air-freighted tender-stem broccoli and sugar-snap peas we have no idea.

All of these overlooked and undercooked ingredients are delicious, sustainable (or reduce waste), and are not difficult to prepare when you know how. They are also pretty cheap in comparison with bland, hormone-stuffed, brine saturated, shrink-wrapped chicken breasts and pork chops.

And that is why we have written this book. We want to convince home cooks that these amazing ingredients are deserving of a place on the plate. This is not just a recipe book or a culinary exploration or even a culinary history: it is a culinary manifesto. It is a declaration of our interest in these ingredients, our affection for these ingredients, and – yes – our love of these ingredients. We want to change the way people think about them and change the way they think about eating them.

Ugly food?

So why don't we eat more octopus? Ironically enough, this was where the journey that led to this book began: we both love eating octopus, and remain utterly bemused by its lack of popularity. When we started looking into it we sensed it was because the octopus has been regarded as a bizarre, mystical and, quite frankly, ugly creature, with a sinister reputation. And what about gurnard and other so-called 'trash fish'? That disparaging term, which we avoid using, says it all: these are fish that are seen as worthless or inferior, in part because some are regarded as just too ugly to eat. Weird ugly root vegetables often suffer a similar fate: cheeks, feet and giblets too. The food industry, like the fashion industry, seems driven by the pursuit of impossible perfection. Endless rows of blemish-free fruit and vegetables in supermarkets that taste of not-very-much. Pre-packaged meats with nary a head or foot or tail in sight. And a steady stream of cookbooks and articles with Photoshopped, super-saturated photos of beautiful dishes bathed in summer sunlight.

Little wonder that we're turned off by a creature with tentacles, suckers and an anus in the middle of its face.

The situation is more complex than that though. For starters, consumers can hardly use ugliness as a justification for refusing to eat rabbit. If anything, rabbits suffer from precisely the opposite problem: they're too darn cute. 'How could you eat a fluffy bunny with floppy ears?' Squirrels are pretty cute too. 'How could anyone eat a sweet, fluffy-tailed, acorn-nibbling squirrel?'

This argument is fatally flawed. Firstly, most people who find rabbits and squirrels too cute to eat wouldn't think twice about sitting down to a lamb chop. Lambs are seriously cute: they gambol; they bleat; we even take our children to pet them and feed them from a bottle. But meat-eaters are happy to eat lamb. Why lambs and not rabbits? Likewise, most non-vegetarians are more than happy to eat bacon. Indeed, many former vegetarians were 'turned' to the dark side by ruthless carnivores grilling bacon the morning after the night before: but, well, have you ever seen *Babe*?

And not only are people perfectly happy to eat ingredients that are, in their natural state, cute; they happily eat ugly ones too! Is a potato good-looking? What about lobsters or oysters? Have you ever looked at a turkey? If George Lucas had populated one of the Star Wars bars with creatures with heads that ugly, fans and critics alike would have said: 'No, you've gone too far this time!'

In reality, it seems that food preferences have little to do with aesthetics. So what's going on? Are people just inconsistent or untruthful?

Probably not. Many people really do justify their refusal to eat certain ingredients on the grounds that they're either too ugly or too cute. But the fact that they avoid ugly fish and rabbit and happily tuck into turkey and lamb suggests that this can't be the real reason. We don't think that they're being disingenuous; rather, it's that people are bad at giving explanations for their preferences and behaviours.

Psychologists have a term for this: the introspection illusion. In a series of experiments in the 1970s, the psychologists Richard Nisbett and Timothy

Wilson showed that we are very confident, but exceedingly bad, at explaining the reasons for our preferences. Further experiments by others shed more light on this. For example, Petter Johansson and colleagues investigated people's insights into their preferences by showing them two photographs of faces and asking which they found more attractive. They were given a closer look at their 'chosen' photograph and asked to verbally explain their choice. However, in some cases the experimenter had swapped the photographs, using sleight of hand. Many people did not notice, but still gave what they thought were genuine explanations of their preference. These must have been unknowingly invented ('confabulated') explanations, because they explain a choice that they never made.

A foodie follow-up experiment involved shoppers in a supermarket tasting two different kinds of jam – spicy cinnamon-apple and bitter grapefruit – then verbally explaining their preference while taking further spoonfuls from the 'chosen' pot. The pots were rigged so that when giving their explanations, the subjects were tasting the jam they had previously rejected. A similar experiment was also done with flavoured teas (pungent Pernod and sweet mango). In each case, most people didn't notice the switch even though the tastes were remarkably different. Yet they continued to express a clear preference for the flavour they didn't choose, and confabulated explanations for their choice.

We all have some pretty deep-seated desires and revulsions – food preferences included. In addition to showing that we're very bad at explaining them, scientists have done a lot of work looking at where they come from. It turns out to be pretty complicated.

There seems to be a range of factors that affect people's food choices. Some revulsions appear to be hard-wired – we don't need to learn to be repulsed by the smell of sewage or the taste of rotting food. We evolved to detect and reject contaminated foods that could cause sickness, and perceived sources of contamination, like cockroaches. Give someone a drink with a cockroach in it, and it's not surprising that they will refuse to drink, even after the cockroach has been removed. Give people a drink that contains a cockroach hermetically sealed in a plastic 'ice-cube', and they will feel physical revulsion – and will probably retch – even though they understand that contamination is impossible.

But these hard-wired reactions are neither totally fixed, nor are they the whole story. Culture and experience have a major impact. They can override hard-wired aversions: we can learn to enjoy bitter coffee, although our bitterness receptors are thought to have evolved to prevent us ingesting toxins. Similarly, childhood exposure can significantly alter the tastes we enjoy or avoid.

And for many children these days, fish means fish fingers and meat means either burgers or nuggets. Cultural perceptions that certain foods are highly prestigious and others low prestige are also important. Interestingly, formerly low prestige foods can often become highly prestigious – former 'working-class' food like oysters and salmon have become prized and celebrated.

Other factors that weigh into our choices include learned information – say, on health scares such as BSE ('mad cow disease'), which may lead us to avoid otherwise favourite dishes such as roast beef on the bone. Medical advice on salt and saturated fats can have a similar effect. Many people cite perceived production ethics as a reason for not eating certain foods, but this is not always consistent: those who refuse to eat foie gras may happily buy eggs from battery hens or intensively-reared chicken.

Ultimately, then, when people say they don't eat rabbits because they're too cute, or octopus because it's too weird, they may be just trying to give voice to a complex set of considerations – not all of them conscious – that influence our food preferences. And in the case of these particular ingredients and the others in this volume, we think much of it has to do with familiarity. If we're not used to seeing certain foods on supermarket shelves or on our plates, we tend to avoid them. This book aims to change that.

A little food philosophy

Neither of us is a professional chef or a restaurateur. But we are committed home cooks and we do have strong feelings and opinions about food. We discovered that when we met at university in London, where we were studying for our PhDs. We both travelled to a conference in Santa Barbara, where we were to present some ideas. The conference proved to be something of a disappointment, but we were delighted to discover that each of us was as obsessive about good food as the other. We learned a great deal on that trip, but not much about language and mental representation. Anyway, we want you the reader to have an idea, from the outset, of what our culinary philosophy is all about. Below we set out our Maxims of Gastronomy: THE MAXIM OF QUALITY, THE MAXIM OF PURITY, THE MAXIM OF AVAILABILITY and THE MAXIM OF SUSTAINABILITY.

Had it not been for our time in academia we would never have even met, and in order to pay homage to this fact we echo here one of the great philosophers of language, Paul Grice. He presented his description of what constitutes rational, cooperative behaviour in the form of a set of 'maxims', but his account is often misconstrued. Critics tend to present his maxims as if they were intended as rules, or even instructions. He intended no such thing, and we ask that you do not misconstrue us in the same way. The maxims that follow are certainly not intended as instructions or orders to you – we have more respect for our readers than that. They merely represent a simple and convenient way of introducing you to our description of the kind of thinking that lies behind successful cooking and happy eating.

The Maxim of Quality

Buy the best produce you can afford. But be aware that this most certainly does not equate with 'buy the most expensive produce you can afford'. Some tender ox cheek from a local butcher (or butchery counter) will be much, much cheaper than a frozen leg of lamb from the other side of the world. Those half-dozen stiff, bright-eyed mackerel or herring on the fishmonger's slab will be much cheaper than the listless, sunken-eyed turbot beside them. A 'prime' ingredient, if it is poor quality, is simply not worth buying. Quality is all, whether you're buying truffles or turnips. Insist on it.

The Maxim of Purity

This is the hardest maxim to pin down. Many years ago, Escoffier came up with his famous dictum. 'Faites simple', he wrote, which Elizabeth David (*French Provincial Cooking*, 1967) translates as 'the avoidance of all unnecessary complication and elaboration' (we are reminded of Grice's own sub-maxim 'Be brief', which he glossed as 'avoid unnecessary prolixity'). We agree with the spirit of the dictum. Needless complication and elaboration is the enemy of good food. However, we find that a lot of nonsense is written about 'simplicity' in food. As the great food-writer and cook Richard Olney once wrote: 'Simplicity – no doubt – is a complex thing' (*Simple French Food*, 1975). Is the simplest way of cooking something the one that uses the least ingredients? Is it the one that uses the least complicated techniques? What precisely does 'simple' mean? Olney discusses this issue at length, and eventually decides that when it comes to cooking the term 'simple' is better replaced with the term 'pure in effect', hence our maxim of purity.

Good food is pure in effect. It tastes of itself. It is food in which flavour combinations work together in harmony. The honest, rustic peasant cooking of Europe, Asia and the Americas is food that is pure in effect. Olney considers *cassoulet* to be an excellent example. *Cassoulet* contains many separate ingredients – mutton, goose, vegetables, Toulouse sausages, wine, herbs and spices – and 'simple' is surely an inappropriate descriptor. Yet the flavours all marry together during the cooking. He describes the final stage of gratinisation as follows:

...a further slow cooking process intermingles all the flavours while a gratin, repeatedly basted, forms, is broken, reforms, is re-broken, a single new savour moving into dominance, cloaking, without destroying, the autonomy of the primitive members.

Replacing the notion of 'simplicity' with that of 'purity in effect allows us also to extol the virtues of the wonderful subtleties of 'Haute Cuisine'. Those who view the great Michelin three-starred kitchens with suspicion (and there are many) argue that the food from such places is 'messed about' or overly complex. But if the aim is to amplify, not alter, the essential basis of the ingredient or dish, then – as *cassoulet* teaches us – a degree of complication is fine. The key word in Elizabeth David's translation of Escoffier's dictum, and a word that is perhaps sometimes overlooked, is 'unnecessary'.

We always try to think about what we're doing. We try not to be lazy. Ingredients must be treated with respect. They can be mixed, but the end result should always be harmonious or 'pure in effect'. This can only be achieved by understanding, and understanding comes through learning.

Imagine you have two fresh sole. What can be the point, as one English culinary deity suggests, in baking them in a sauce made of mashed broccoli mixed with a supermarket-bought leek and Gruyère cheese sauce? Only one: to disguise the taste of the fish. But we have followed the MAXIM OF QUALITY. Our fish smell of the sea. They are firm to the touch, and their eyes are not sunken – they are positively staring back at us (this is one of our top tips for choosing fresh fish). So just season them lightly and grill them, or sauté them in clarified butter and serve sprinkled with parsley. The purity of effect can be enhanced, maybe with the addition of a few capers, or a scrap of garlic, or a squeeze of lemon. If it's a special occasion, then bake the fish with a few drops of white vermouth, into which you mix some double cream just before serving. Use your imagination, yes, but move in the direction of harmony, not cacophony.

THE MAXIM OF AVAILABILITY

Cook with what is seasonal and – as far as possible – with what is local. (And we choose local over organic any day.) We don't try and impress our friends with *that* dish from *that* glossy cookbook if the ingredients aren't in season and aren't available locally. Of course, the word 'local' is a tricky one. Your 'local' supermarket may well sell frozen Cambodian prawns, but that doesn't count (unless you live in Phnom Penh). A restaurant local to one of us on the south coast of England prides itself on serving 'local', fresh seafood. Yet the menu features 'Isle of Lewis mussels' and 'Loch Fyne Queenie scallops'. The Outer Hebrides are more than 750 miles from this restaurant. It's therefore closer to Marseille in the South of France, than it is to the source of its mussels. And this restaurant is less than 20 metres from the sea.

Such an approach to sourcing ingredients suggests laziness, and not only violates the Maxim of Availability, but the two previous maxims also. Freshly shucked, the quality of south coast scallops is unsurpassable. Seared in a little oil and served with garlic butter, or some lardons of bacon and salad leaves, they are the epitome of purity.

But one should certainly not be dogmatic about this. The world is getting smaller, and the sheer quality of certain ingredients, from certain places, renders the issue of locality almost irrelevant. These ingredients are fantastic because of where they are from, and they are widely available simply because of their quality.

Think of the French concept of *terroir*. There is no literal English translation, but the general idea is that there is a unique, symbiotic relationship between a specific ingredient and the geographical location in which it is produced (and everything that might involve – the landscape, the climate, the soil, the human activity). The term is often used in discussion of wine. Those heady, sun-filled red wines of the South of France are the perfect expression of the long, baking summers in which the grapes grow. By contrast the crisp, dry whites of the Loire are the embodiment of the flinty chalky soil of the Loire Valley and the cool winter air that blows through it. We buy Spanish saffron, though neither of us lives in Spain. We grate parmesan cheese on our (Italian) pasta, and adore Parma ham, though neither of us lives in Parma. There is a good reason for buying these non-local ingredients; frozen fish or meat from the other side of the world is a very different story.

The Maxim of Sustainability

This final maxim is critical. There is currently no agreed definition of what makes food 'sustainable' ('Sustain: the alliance for better food and farming' define sustainability according to four guidelines, which you can find on their website.) However, common sense dictates that at the heart of any such definition there will be at least two requirements. Firstly, the production of food must not damage, waste or destroy natural resources. For a prime example of what has been, and arguably still is, an entirely non-sustainable food practice, just take a look at the sea-fishing industry. The sea is being over-exploited. Stocks of certain fish are critically endangered. If we don't stop fishing them, these fish will become commercially extinct – some already are. There is no getting away from this, and we should all be finding ways to minimise the impact.

Secondly, and perhaps less obviously, practices can surely not be regarded as sustainable unless they protect not only the diversity and well-being of the natural world, but also the welfare and general well-being of farmed and wild animals. Battery chicken farming is now illegal in the UK, but to meet the massive demand for cheap chicken and cheap eggs elsewhere in the EU, there are – according to the organisation Compassion in World Farming – currently over 300 million chickens living in tiny cages; the situation for some farmed rabbits is no better. It's as completely unnecessary as it is barbaric. It has to stop, and it's up to us (all of us) to make sure it does.

The core techniques

How important is a knowledge of cooking technique? We are both self-taught cooks, and we are aware that our cooking has developed not by trial and error (though that has probably played a role), nor by miraculous leaps of creativity, but by reading about food from serious food writers (Elizabeth David, Edouard de Pomiane) as well as serious chefs (Thomas Keller, Raymond Blanc). We have learned, slowly, that most recipes revolve around one – or sometimes more than one – 'core' technique, and that this technique might be applied to a wide range of different ingredients. Having these core techniques in your repertoire means that whatever ingredients you are faced with, you are never completely in the dark: you always have a recipe in your head that will stand you in good stead.

'But if it's all about techniques and recipes…', we hear you ask, '… what about those amazing cooks who say they never follow recipes?' We think such people fall into two separate camps. In the first are those who refuse to follow recipes and genuinely just 'throw' things together. They regard themselves as too darn creative to get down and dirty with anything as limiting as someone else's recipe. Well, yes. But how many such people really are amazing cooks? More often than not they are the only ones who enjoy the fruits of their labours. We suggest that you never throw things together. On the rare occasions that the 'throw-it-all-together' approach does pay dividends, it only does so by chance. If you've spent time and money sourcing great ingredients, why leave turning them into a delicious meal to chance?

What people in the second camp generally mean when they say they don't follow recipes is that they don't necessarily have a set of directions or instructions written down in front of them when they cook. It's the same when famous chefs say things such as – 'Recipes? No. I just follow my instincts' (the kind of claim that is enough to make any amateur cook want to give up). Remember that the chef who is simply 'following their instincts' is using years, perhaps decades, of experience, during which time they have never stopped adapting and honing techniques they acquired during their training and during the course of their day-to-day preparation and cooking of food.

Of course, this is not to say some people don't have a flair for cooking, in the same way that some people have a flair for playing the piano. Some chefs are incredibly talented and imaginative. But the importance of technique should not be underestimated. If you don't believe us, go and ask a professional pianist if they ever practise.

We happily admit that, when we need to, we work directly from a recipe in a cookbook. You should too. If you're attempting to make an authentic dish from a cuisine you are not familiar with; using a complex mixture of herbs, spices and other unfamiliar ingredients, you'd be unwise not to. The same goes for baking cakes, or making patisserie, where precision with quantities is integral to the success of the final dish. But having said that, we often – probably more often than not – cook without a written recipe in front of us. It might look as if we aren't following a recipe, and it might look as if we don't need one, but – believe us – we are following a recipe in our head. We'd never work without one. Of course it's true that as amateurs we lack professional experience, but that doesn't mean an understanding of some of the basic, core techniques of cookery is beyond us. We may never achieve the breadth of knowledge, depth of understanding or sheer competence in difficult techniques of someone who works with food 24/7. But we can aspire.

And – let's face it – we have all eaten food cooked in restaurants by 'professionals' knowing perfectly well we could have done better ourselves. In the chapters that follow we'll not just provide individual recipes, we'll also introduce you to a range of core techniques, which means you will always have that recipe in your head. Typically, these reflect a technique we believe to be important in mastering the cooking of the particular ingredient or set of ingredients that we are focusing on. Each chapter also has 'hack boxes': simple, quick, easy things you can do to cook better with the ingredients in this book or make your life easier in the kitchen.

The recipes themselves are specifically designed to be ones that you can build on in interesting ways. Indeed, rather than simply reading and slavishly following any of the recipes in this book, we'd like to think that you will use the ideas in them as points of departure, from which you can embark on your own culinary journeys and explorations. As just one example, take the recipe for beef in red wine (Daube de boeuf Bourguignon) on page 66 in the **Cheeks and Feet** chapter. The core technique (or set of core techniques, depending on how you look at it) behind this recipe might roughly be summarised as follows:

- Marinate the meat for a time.
- Brown it well in fat.
- Remove the meat and brown the vegetables also.

- Add the meat back to the pan with the marinade and some other cooking medium, and cook slowly, slowly, slowly.

As we point out after the recipe, there are a number of ways it might be built upon. Let's begin with the meat. You could replace the ox cheeks with pigs cheeks, or lamb shanks, or sheep trotters, or any other meat that is suitable for slow cooking. You might even mix your cuts: it would make sense to include some belly pork with your pigs' cheek, and maybe a trotter or two, for extra unctuousness. If you do this, you may also want to think about changing the liquid in which your meat is to be cooked – perhaps white wine, or cider? If you have got your hands on some chorizo, that would make a perfect addition. But always keep the maxims in mind. If that's the direction your dish is heading, then know that while a teaspoon of *pimenton* would also make sense, a teaspoon of curry powder would not.

You may also want to use a different selection of vegetables. Leek will add a lovely, gentle allium flavour to any stew; fennel will give it a subtle aniseed background. And while the dish is hardly one for hot weather, if summer has begun to turn to autumn and you still have access to some deliciously ripe plum tomatoes, add them (perhaps with a bundle of herbs you have snipped from a friend's garden). Some soaked (or even tinned) chickpeas or haricot beans would also work well. You get the picture.

We'd also encourage you to feel confident enough to carry over recipes from one chapter to ingredients that feature in another. The octopus rice dish on page 44 works equally well with anglerfish, one of the ugliest fish of all; the recipe for Arroz a Banda in the chapter Ugly Fish would be delightful if accompanied by some braised octopus. The Daube de boeuf Bourguignon works beautifully with rabbit (though make sure you alter the cooking time accordingly) and, for that matter, the Hearty Rabbit Soup on page 161 would be even heartier if enriched with a trotter or two. Our recipe for Goose Giblets with Root Vegetables on page 250 works as nicely with celeriac and mangel-wurzel as it does with more commonly used root vegetables included in our recipe; a few strands of slow cooked ox-cheek added to the recipe for Burdock *Kinpira Style* on page 210 turn a light vegetable accompaniment into a full meal.

So feel free to experiment, but at the same time respect the maxims: Quality – buy the best you can afford; Purity – always move in the direction of harmony, not cacophony; Availability – shop seasonally and locally; Sustainability – make your shopping, and your lifestyle, sustainable.

Cook ugly food!

It's beautiful.

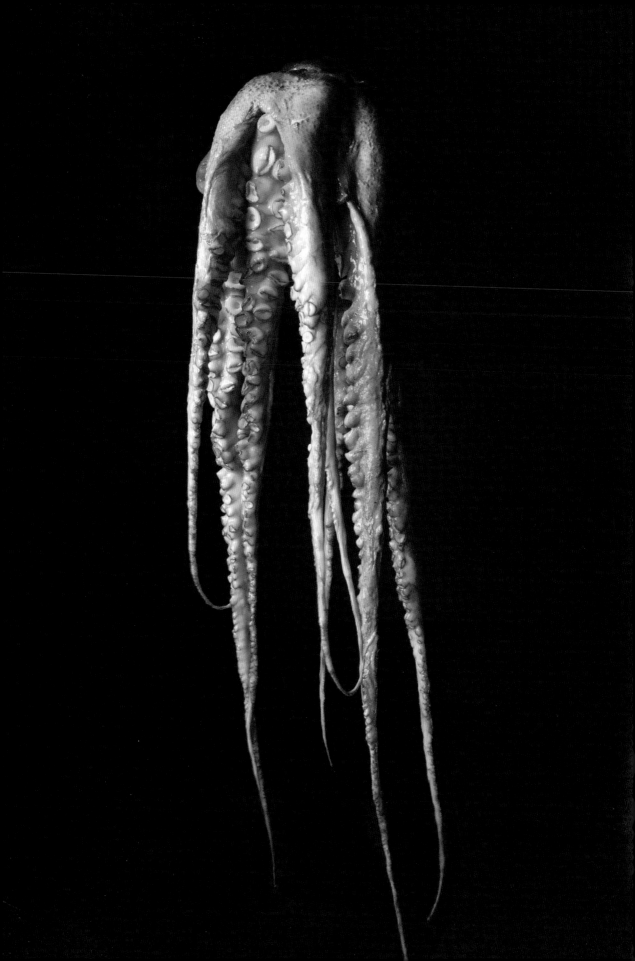

2. OCTOPUS

The kraken wakes

Octopus can be prepared in so many ways. It can be braised in a pressure cooker or boiled in liquid, the arms then separated from the body, or 'mantle'. Take some of the chopped up arms and prepare a spicy and refreshing Vietnamese Octopus Salad (on page 37) with lemongrass, cucumber and onion, or serve them in a warming Arroz do Polvo (on page 44), a kind of Portuguese octopus risotto with tomato, red pepper and the juices that have seeped out of the octopus in the pressure cooker. You can charcoal grill, or place on a dry cast-iron griddle, until they develop charred stripes that lend the flesh a rich smoky flavour, and eat them as an appetiser like the Greeks do – with salt and olive oil, or even as a main meal with some boiled potatoes. Perhaps you'd prefer an octopus curry from the Maldives or a *daube* of octopus from Provence? And don't forget the mantle. This can be thinly sliced and dressed with a lemon, herb and garlic dressing – perhaps with a few cockles, prawns or mussels.

Why don't people eat octopus? That's one of the things this chapter is about. Why are British shoppers simply not interested in the humble, yet delicious octopus? In Japan, for example, *tako i*s a delicacy, which features in a range of amazing dishes. And many countries in continental Europe eat huge quantities of octopus: France, Greece, Italy, Portugal, Spain, Turkey, to name but a few.

If octopus is tasty, cheap and sustainable, then what of its legendary toughness? Surely it must be difficult to cook correctly? We disagree. Ignore everything you've read about the need for elaborate tenderisation before cooking. It's simply not true. Cooked correctly you'll find that no tenderisation is necessary; cooked incorrectly, you're likely to end up with tough, rubbery octopus no matter how many times you've beaten it on a rock or how many wine corks you've boiled it with. And if you don't believe us, just give it a try – once you know how, you'll find it's much, much more difficult to make octopus tough than it is to make it tender. Cooking octopus is really very easy once you know the basic principles, and in the pages that follow, we'll show you how.

We want to convince you that the octopus is an amazing creature in so many different ways. Once you have finished this chapter, we hope that you will not only know a great deal more about the octopus, but you will also experiment freely and regularly with this wonderfully tasty and economical ingredient.

Poulpe fictions

DEVILFISH

In Victor Hugo's sweeping novel *Toilers of the Sea* the hero – Gilliatt – attempts against all the odds to salvage the engines of the *Durande*, a steamer that has run aground on a treacherous reef between the coasts of Guernsey and Brittany. In doing so he pits himself not only against the vertiginous cliffs that frame the reef, a raging storm, driving rain, vicious currents and unpredictable surging tides, but also the devilfish or *pieuvre* – the Guernsey-French word that Hugo's book helped re-establish into the French vernacular largely at the expense of the word *poulpe*.

It is, according to Hugo, an abominable creature:

> All ideals being valid, if causing terror is an objective, then the devilfish is a masterpiece. ... The devilfish has no mass of muscle, no threatening cry, no armour, no horn, no sting, no pincers, no tail to seize or hold its enemies, no sharp-edged fins, no clawed-fins, no spines, no sword, no electric discharge, no poison, no claws, no beak, no teeth. And yet of all animals the devilfish is that one that is most formidably armed. What, then, is the devilfish? It is a suction pad. ...

> This monster is the creature that seamen call the octopus, scientists call a cephalopod, and which in legend is known as a kraken. English sailors call it the devilfish or bloodsucker. In the Channel Islands it is called the *pieuvre*.

As well as being a wonderful writer, Hugo was an accomplished artist. Buy *Toilers of the Sea*, or do an online search, and enjoy his eerie, brooding illustrations of the beast.

To readers of the 1860s Hugo's *pieuvre* was what Peter Benchley's man-eater in *Jaws* was to readers of the 1970s: a cold-blooded monster which existed merely to kill. *Toilers of the Sea* arguably did as much for the public relations of the beloved cephalopod as Peter Benchley's book – and the subsequent box-office smash film – did for the Great White shark.

The devilfish is pure evil:

...the octopus has all human passions: it can hate. And indeed, in the absolute to be hideous is to hate. ...

It has only one orifice, in the centre, from which the tentacles radiate. Is this single opening the anus? Is it the mouth? Is it both? The same opening serves both functions. The entrance is also the exit.

The whole creature is cold.

A year after the publication of *Toilers*, an octopus was put on display in the aquarium in Boulogne, France. Four years after that, in 1871, Crystal Palace Aquarium in London advertised its own devilfish, and hordes of curious punters queued in the grounds before parting with their sixpences (threepence for children) to see the beast. Victorian aquaria expert J. E. Taylor wrote:

Victor Hugo, in his *Toilers of the Sea*, had prepared the public mind...; and accordingly the first specimen of a living octopus in the Crystal Palace Aquarium had to bear the uninterrupted gaze of lookers-on for weeks. It sat for its portrait in the illustrated papers, and had all its points noted down by newspaper correspondents with the same faithful detail as if they were those of prize cattle at the Agricultural Show.

Henry Lee, a Victorian naturalist, caused Benchley-esque levels of panic among beach-goers on the south coast of England when he reported that the octopus that became an exhibit at Brighton Aquarium the year after the Crystal Palace event, had actually been caught in a lobster-pot in Eastbourne, just a few miles down the coast.

Earlier this year in an episode right out of *Finding Nemo*, Inky, a Common New Zealand octopus living in the National Aquarium of New Zealand in Napier, managed to escape to freedom in the waters surrounding New Zealand's North Island. According to the aquarium's own account, the lid of Inky's pen was left slightly ajar overnight. On realising this, Inky crawled to the top, escaped down the side and slid across the aquarium floor to the mouth of a drainpipe leading direct to the sea. The drainpipe is 50 metres long, so Inky's journey would have been far from straightforward. However, as we'll see later, not only are octopuses prodigiously intelligent creatures, they are also incredible contortionists.

And yes, we say octopuses, not 'octopi'. Strictly speaking, the plural ending 'i' is only used with words ending in 'us' that are etymologically Latin. Octopus (in common with platypus) is etymologically Greek. But we're pretty relaxed linguists and genuinely have no axe to grind over this: so say what you want. Actually, we find it pretty objectionable that the 2004 edition of the *Cambridge Guide to English Usage* finds use of the word octopi 'objectionable'. You'll notice also that we refer to octopus 'arms': the term 'tentacle' is generally reserved for the pair of elongated limbs that squid and cuttlefish have in addition to their eight arms.

To return to the work of Hugo and Benchley, they of course knew precisely what they were doing. A fear of the deep sea and the mysterious creatures which live there – or don't live there – is pretty much universal and writers, painters, photographers and filmmakers play on that. It may well be that the fear is programmed into humans. The 'snake-fear' reflex is widely accepted as an innately determined part of human psychological make-up; it has served us well as a species to be frightened of snakes and we are hard-wired to be this way. Those of our early human ancestors who avoided venomous snakes were the ones who lived to reproduce. A fear of the deep – known as thalassophobia – may also come from our primordial brains.

Recent work in evolutionary psychology suggests that the human capacity for superstition is also an evolved trait, one that has developed in our species as a way of rationalising what we simply don't understand. Where the facts are missing, we create fictions. Then within a community or culture, stories that reflect these fictions are told, retold, and spread to become beliefs. Folklore and mythology develop in this way. In many cultures, children are introduced to these fictions as facts about the world.

Hugo's book is full of the local Guernsey folk's beliefs in ghosts, witches and the Devil. So as well as an underlying fear of the deep sea, the human disposition to interpret the unknown in terms of superstition and myth probably provided even more fertile ground in which Hugo could plant the seeds of terror. He continues:

> These animals are phantoms as much as monsters. … You deny the existence of the vampire, and the octopus appears.

Hugo, however, was not on some one-man anti-octopus crusade. In his defence, the creature's reputation was hardly unblemished before his novel. Whilst Tennyson's 'kraken' does not feature by name in the Norse sagas, sea monsters matching its description most definitely do. The *hafgufa* was a huge creature, which lived on the sea floor and was fed constantly by attendant fish. In these sagas the *hafgufa* is always distinguishable from other sea monsters, such as serpents and dragons, and there are tales of its ability to drag whole ships down to the ocean floor, as well as of the terrifying whirlpools it caused when it headed back down to the depths. In the seventeenth century, the Swedish Bishop of Uppsala Olaus Magnus reported that he had spoken to fishermen who claimed to have encountered kraken with 50-yard-long tentacles. Whereas in his natural history of the area, the Norwegian bishop Pontoppidan writes that when it comes to the surface from its deep-sea lair, the kraken – by this time the name was in use – is approximately two and a half miles in diameter.

Now that is one giant octopus.

It's arguable that the Norse sagas may not have been the first to feature creatures inspired by the octopus. While the deadly *scylla* in the *Odyssey* was described by Homer as having six heads and twelve feet, his description of the creature resting with its back in a cave, and reaching out with its tentacle-like arms/legs in order to eat anything that passes, suggests that the octopus may have been the inspiration behind the creature. Living among the Greek Islands, as it is claimed he did, Homer would have encountered octopuses on a regular basis (though normally on a plate).

Some sixty years before Hugo's book, and inspired by the discovery of a two and a half metre tentacle in the mouth of a sperm whale, French naturalist Pierre Denys de Montfort wrote of the 'kraken octopus' in his *Histoire naturelle générale et particulière des mollusques*. This, he claimed, was the terrifying sea monster that American whalers and North European mariners had given accounts of, and which was implicated in the disappearance of many ships and the deaths of countless seamen. De Montfort's illustration 'Colossal Octopus' shows the grotesqueness and awesome destructive power of the creature. The fact that eighteenth- and nineteenth-century writers and artists linked their mythological sea creatures with the octopus is probably largely due to the fact that in his seminal tome *Systema Naturae*, Carl Linnaeus – the father of modern biological taxonomy – classified the kraken as a cephalopod. In later editions, however, the kraken was omitted.

De Montfort's work was dismissed by his fellow academics, who regarded the existence of giant cephalopods as nothing more than an old wives' tale. And he was totally discredited when the Royal Navy refuted his claim that ten British ships sunk in 1782 must have been attacked and destroyed by giant octopuses. The Navy knew precisely what had happened to the ships, and confirmed that no such creatures were involved. It was not until some forty years later, and just a few years before Hugo's novel was published, that the existence of the kind of giant sea monster de Montfort described gained acceptance among scientists. The kraken does exist. Unfortunately for de Montfort, who died in abject poverty, it isn't a giant octopus. It's a giant squid.

As far as we know.

Octopus's Garden

I think it's great that you've got eight wobbly arms
I can never see you with your crazy camouflage
I think your bostin!
You are surreal!
Better than the fish the sharks and even the conger eel!

'Octopus I love you', Dalmatian Rex and the Eigentones

While psychedelically-coloured octopuses cavort jollily in the Beatles' wonderful animated film *Yellow Submarine*, Ringo's classic tune 'Octopus's Garden' actually appeared on 'Abbey Road', the album that followed. Ringo's songs were always popular with children, and it's interesting to compare the playful octopus of his song (and that of legendary Leicester band Dalmatian Rex), and indeed children's films and books, with the menacing, deathly presence of Hugo's illustration and de Montfort's pseudo-science. Think back to the octopus that plays drums (whilst simultaneously dealing cards) in *Bedknobs and Broomsticks*, or the octopus Dr Dolittle asks for directions in the famous 1967 film. Go and peruse the shelves in the children's section of your local bookshop. Among the books you may find will be *Tickly Octopus* or *Gentle Giant Octopus*, or *Octopus Socktopus* or *Jolly Olly Octopus* or *The Friendly Octopus*. You may even find *My Very Own Octopus*, a book published in 1991 that features on the cover a small boy, cheerfully entangled in the tentacles of a smiling octopus. This last cover is – to our minds – more terrifying than anything Hugo could have dreamt up.

But when it comes to mainstream popular entertainment, Ringo's happy, lilting 'We all live in a yellow submarine...' melody must fade quickly away, and be replaced by much more appropriate slow, brooding chords (think the bowed double-bass soundtrack to *Jaws* and you're halfway there). The history of the octopus in mainstream film is similar to that in mainstream literature. It's a monster. It's evil. It's death. On the covers of aptly named 'pulp' comic books, the octopus is always a villain and, interestingly enough, enjoys a diet that consists mainly of scantily-clad women. (For wonderful pulp comic book covers we highly recommend Francesca Myman's personal website at francesca.net/pulp.html).

Ray Friedgen's 1937 film *Killers of the Sea* relates in pseudo-documentary format the story of Captain Wallace Caswell Jr. This Florida Chief of Police is determined to protect the game fish of the Gulf of Mexico. As well as protecting them from illegal poachers, he also declares war on natural marine predators that have (fairly legitimately, you would think) moved into the Gulf to feed on the bounty. The premise is unthinkable today and some of the humour is downright racist – listen to the narrator's mimicking of 'Evolution' Henderson, the ship's cook – but among those evil predators that meet their end at Caswell's hands (quite literally) are sharks, whales, dolphins, turtles and – you've guessed it – an octopus. The film is a monochrome gore-fest. And if you're beginning to think the title of the film is ironic, things are more complex than you may think. Caswell was a real person, and he really was proudly known as the 'Killer of the Sea'.

In the climax to the 1954 film *Beneath the Twelve Mile Reef*, also set off the coast of Florida, a young sponge diver played by Robert Wagner finds an underwater cave that is full of sponges. The only problem is that the cave is also home to a giant octopus. Wagner grapples the octopus and – to the huge relief of fans of *Hart to Hart* – emerges the winner. For those interested in such trivia, when Wagner's character stabs the octopus, it bleeds red blood. Oxygenated octopus blood, as we shall learn later in this chapter, is blue.

There are many other films featuring octopus villains. In the James Bond film *Octopussy* the baddies are tattooed with blue-ringed octopuses. Davy Jones, one of the main protagonists in *Pirates of the Caribbean: Dead Man's Chest*, is portrayed as an eerie part-human, part-cephalopod creature, with a 'beard' of octopus tentacles. Jones's beard arguably pays homage to the alien creature Cthulhu from H.P. Lovecraft's horror books of the 1920s. That classic cult film maker Edward Wood Jr. (think *Plan 9 from Outer Space*) made a film starring the wonderful Bela Lugosi as a mad scientist who possesses a giant octopus that – miraculously – lives in a freshwater lake. Some species of octopus can survive for a while in brackish water, but freshwater kills them.

By far our favourite on-screen octopus, however, is the star of the 1977 film *Tentacles*. The film attracted some big names – Henry Fonda, John Huston and Shelley Winters – but was a box-office flop. The story revolves around a seaside resort, Ocean Beach, which is being terrorised by a huge beast that attacks bathers, and leaves their skeletons picked absolutely clean of all flesh. Naturally, as the number of attacks increase, so tourists are discouraged from visiting the resort. (If the story sounds vaguely familiar, *Tentacles* came out two years after *Jaws* and was presumably an effort to cash in on its success.) In the climax to the film the beast, which turns out to be an enraged giant octopus, is killed by two trained killer whales.

Poulpe fictions indeed. Time for some facts.

Poulpe facts

The octopus really has got a bad press over the years, entirely undeservedly. In setting the record straight, you will find that the facts are even more remarkable than the fiction. Although these creatures are molluscs (think snails and mussels), the differences could hardly be more striking. Here are twelve things you probably didn't know about the enigmatic octopus.

1. Octopuses have three hearts that pump blue blood. Two hearts are dedicated to pumping blood through the two gills, while the third takes care of the body. Octopus blood is blue because it transports oxygen not using iron-rich haemoglobin (which turns red when oxygenated), but rather the copper-rich protein haemocyanin (which turns blue when oxygenated).

2. Octopuses are incredible contortionists. With no skeleton or shell, not even the 'bone' of its cuttlefish cousin, the only hard part of an octopus is its beak. This enables it to squeeze through extremely small cracks – very useful for hiding and hunting on a coral reef. Octopuses have been found living in beer bottles – able to squeeze their bodies through the narrow neck of the bottle – and have even been known to escape from their aquariums through the water pipes.

3. Octopuses move in mysterious ways. Their slowest and most common approach is crawling along the seabed using the suckers on their arms to pull themselves along. But when necessary they can move backwards with remarkable velocity and acceleration using jet propulsion – sucking water into their mantle and using its powerful muscles to expel the water quickly through the funnel, which can be rotated to point them in the desired direction. They can also swim forwards in a similar manner, but more slowly, with the funnel facing the opposite way. The veined octopus (*O. marginatus*) from Indonesia can even walk in a bipedal fashion on two of its arms while using the rest to disguise itself as a coconut.

4. Octopuses are fearsome predators. When a giant octopus was moved into a large display tank at the Seattle aquarium that also contained sharks, staff were a little concerned for its safety. But then shark carcasses started turning up at the bottom of the tank. Video footage showed that the octopus was ambushing and eating the sharks.

5. All octopuses are venomous. In addition to their powerful arms, octopuses have a number of other tools for dealing with prey. They have a hard parrot-like beak for crushing food or breaking open shells and a toothed tongue (the radula) used for drilling into shells or scraping out food. But they are also equipped with a fang-like gland (the salivary papilla) that can inject a toxic saliva that paralyses and partially digests prey – a favourite octopus trick is to inject this saliva into the eye of a crab, rapidly immobilising it. Although all octopuses have these nerve toxins, only the tiny golf-ball-size blue-ringed octopus is potentially deadly to humans, with enough toxin to kill twenty-six people.

6. *Octopuses are highly intelligent.* They may very well be the smartest of all invertebrates, although just how such an ability evolved in an animal related to slugs and clams remains something of a mystery. They have individual personalities, engage in play and can learn to navigate mazes, open jars and bottles, and recognise different people. It has recently been shown that they also engage in tool-use, a rare trait in the animal kingdom that is considered a mark of high intelligence. The ability to predict football matches is not normally considered so highly by intelligence researchers, but in the 2010 World Cup, one octopus named Paul proved curiously accurate at doing so. Paul's predictions were so influential that bookmakers Paddy Power reported that they were turning the global betting market on its head; the German aquarium that owned him rejected a 100,000 Euro offer from a Russian gambling syndicate and quickly announced his retirement.

7. *Octopuses are masters of disguise.* Their skin is covered with thousands of chromatophores – independently controllable pigment cells that can change colour in less than a second – allowing them to blend into their surroundings with stunning accuracy. They can even change the texture of their skin to further improve their camouflage. Some octopuses combine their flexibility and colour-changing skills to imitate other creatures such as sea snakes or lionfish, to deter potential predators. And if camouflage or mimicry doesn't work, they can squirt a cloud of ink that hides their escape, and also contains compounds that interfere with the predator's sense of smell and taste.

8. *Some species of octopus can wilfully detach one of their arms,* which slithers off as an enticing decoy for predators. This is an ability known as 'autotomy'; the amputated arm can be regenerated. Amputated arms literally have minds of their own: unlike mammals, the octopus nervous system is distributed, with three-fifths of its neurones in the arms. This also explains why detached arms can readily choke Korean diners, on which more later.

9. *Octopuses can create replicas of themselves from ink.* When threatened, some octopuses can make decoys by squirting mucous-laden clouds of ink of about the same size and appearance as the octopus (called 'pseudomorphs'). As they do this, they change their own colour, causing the predator to attack the decoy.

10. *Octopuses live fast and die young.* They grow very quickly, reproduce only once, and then become demented ('senescent') and die shortly

afterwards – males within a few months of mating, and females once their eggs hatch. This gives octopuses surprisingly short lifespans – typically, between one and three years.

11. *Some octopuses have detachable penises.* During reproduction, the male of some species breaks off his sperm-laden arm (a form of autotomy, see 8.) and gives it to the female, who stores it in her mantle. Later, once she has laid her eggs, she takes out the arm and spreads the sperm it holds over the eggs. Nineteenth century naturalists who came across these mobile 'penises' inside octopus females can be forgiven for not fathoming their true nature; they believed they were parasitic worms.

12. *Octopus wrestling was once a very popular sport in the United States.* It became so popular in the 1960s that annual World Octopus Wrestling Championships were held. After being wrestled, octopuses were released, eaten, or given to local aquariums. According to a 1965 issue of *Time* magazine: 'although there are several accepted techniques for octopus wrestling, the really sporty way requires that the human diver go without artificial breathing apparatus'.

SPECIES OF CULINARY INTEREST

The word 'octopus' in English is ambiguous, referring broadly to creatures in the order *Octopoda*, or just in the family *Octopodidae*, or in a narrow sense only to those of the genus *Octopus*. In this book, we are generally using the term in the middle sense, to refer to the family *Octopodidae* – which contains most of the familiar, bottom-dwelling octopuses, including all of the important culinary species. And it means that in discussing the physiology and behaviour of octopuses, we are not thinking of unusual creatures like the Dumbo octopuses – a family of charming deep-sea octopuses with a pair of large fins that look like elephant ears.

Classifying octopuses can get pretty confusing, as there are over a hundred species in the genus *Octopus* alone. Also, certain classifications are controversial – and not just those of unusual or recently-discovered creatures. There is a long-running debate among scientists regarding the common octopus (*O. vulgaris*), which is regarded as a 'cryptic species complex' – not, as you might imagine, a curious form of marine paranoia, but a technical way of saying that scientists suspect the common octopus is actually several different species, but that they don't know how to tell them apart.

Many species of octopus around the world are caught for food – either as a targeted catch, or as by-catch. Given the global nature of the seafood industry, there's really no telling which species might turn up in your local market. But, as always, we'd encourage you to ask your fishmonger, and try to stick with local produce as much as possible. Here are some of the varieties you are more likely to come across.

O. vulgaris species complex ('common octopus')

> The common octopus (*O. vulgaris*) is the one that you are most likely to find at your local fishmongers, although many other species may be encountered. But don't always believe what you are told, particularly if the octopus is not sourced locally: since there are numerous species that look very similar, even to experts, the seafood industry often labels them simply as 'octopus' – and some suppliers misleadingly label all species as '*O. vulgaris*'.

Found in temperate and tropical waters worldwide, most commonly in shallower coastal areas. In the Atlantic, found up to the south coast of the UK, Virginia in the US, and Bermuda. Can be active both during the day and at night. It is estimated that around 100,000 tonnes are taken each year, accounting for about half of the global octopus catch. Grows to a total length of 130 cm, and commonly weighs up to 3 kg (although it can reach 10 kg). Each arm has two rows of suckers.

O. macropus species complex ('white-spotted octopus')

Found in tropical and warm-temperate seas, typically in shallow coastal waters. It has long arms (the front two being longer than the rest) with shallow webbing, and a higher number of suckers than most other octopuses, arranged in two rows. It is predominantly nocturnal and smaller than the common octopus, growing to a total length of 80 cm and weighing up to 2 kg. Several other species are very similar, at least from a culinary point of view, including the quite large Maori octopus, *O. maorum,* and the smaller southern or hammer octopus, *O. australis* – the most common species caught off the east coast of Australia.

Eledone cirrhosa ('curled octopus'; sometimes referred to as the 'lesser octopus')

Octopuses in the genus *Eledone* are distinguished by having only a single row of suckers on each arm. The name 'curled octopus' refers to the fact that when at rest, the ends of its arms curl up. These octopuses are widely eaten, and can be very tasty, but they are often rather small, and their flavour and texture is somewhat inferior to that of *O. vulgaris*. A very similar species, *E. moschata*, the 'musky octopus', is common in the Mediterranean. It gets its name from the fact that it emits a strong musky odour when pulled from the water.

Other sub-species

There is a range of other sub-species that are often eaten: *Cistopus indicus* ('old woman octopus'); *O. cyanea* ('big blue octopus'); *O. aegina* species complex ('marbled octopus'); and the largest of them all, *Enteroctopus dofleini* and *magnificus* ('giant octopus'). Giant octopuses typically grow to a total length of 2–4 metres. They commonly weigh between 2 kg and 10 kg, but specimens of *E. dofleini* weighing over 50 kg have been recorded. Their thick arms are particularly prized for sushi.

To get a sense of just how big they can be, consider the smallish specimen below (for scale, that is a 20 cm chef's knife, 34 cm including the handle). One of us, who was living in southern Africa at the time, ordered a large box of frozen octopus when doing some recipe development for this book, and discovered after thawing it in the sink that the consignment consisted of just two specimens – this one and another that was of a similar size. We are pleased to report that after braising it according to our method below, it was beautifully tender.

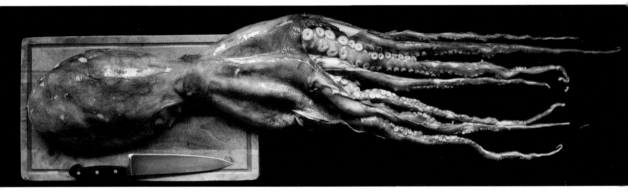

A typical *E. magnificus* specimen. This one was 130 cm long and weighed 7 kg.

Octopuses have a global distribution, and it is hardly surprising that they are part of the culinary traditions of many cultures around the world. They are a staple food in the Mediterranean, north Africa, South America, the Pacific islands, and much of Asia. What is surprising is that they have been largely ignored by Anglo-American food culture, despite their ready availability off the coasts of the UK and US. And this is not just a recent phenomenon: octopus doesn't appear in traditional British recipe books – there is no mention, for example, in Dorothy Hartley's seminal *Food in England*.

In fact, we may have to go back to Roman times to find the last time octopus was popular in Britain. With their keen eye for the bizarre as well as the delicious, the Romans were very partial to octopus. It appeared in many of their mosaics, and as a food they attributed to it the power of restoring lost vitality. But even they seemed to go as much for shock value as taste, using boiled octopus as a dining-table centrepiece – the mass of pink arms suggestive of a fearsome creature from the deep. The Roman culinary text *Apicius* gives this rather short recipe:

> For octopus:
> pepper, liquamen [salty fermented fish sauce] and laser [asafoetida]. Serve.

The tendency to prize octopus for its combination of shock value and imputed restorative powers persists to this day. Notoriously, Korean diners eat live octopus (either whole, or one tentacle at a time for the larger specimens), a dangerous practice that sometimes results in death by choking from the wriggling arms. Some Koreans – particularly practitioners of the martial art Kendo – believe that eating live octopus helps to build strength and stamina. Or maybe it's just a macho thing. The grandmotherly advice to chew well before swallowing is particularly pertinent here; it could save your life.

As for Americans, well one traveller to Samoa in the 1930s was offered octopus, and described it as 'the worst thing I ever nerved myself to try'. A few spoonfuls made him 'violently sick', and this despite a later admission that he learned to like very well a local dish of sea worms that resembled tapeworms. He describes the octopus recipe as follows:

> First, take a live and squirming octopus of about moderate size and drop it into the stew pot. The real essence of the stew is lost if the ink has been drained from the ink sac. If this is lost, it is best to throw the octopus away and get a new one. Then add two gallons of coconut milk and the juice of six limes to every ten pounds of octopus. Stir well but make sure that the octopus does not wrench the ladle from your hands or crawl out of the pot. The water is kept boiling with hot rocks until the octopus is quite thoroughly dead. The stew is then considered ready to serve. Serve it hot, garnished with a dash of finely grated tobacco leaves.
>
> Donald Sloan, *The Shadow Catcher*, New York: Book League of America, 1940

But no discussion of strange octopus dishes would be complete without mentioning Japanese octopus balls. And before you get carried away, we should tell you that this refers to the shape of the final dish. According to media reports, octopus balls, or *takoyaki*, were first made in 1935 in south Osaka as a variation on traditional dumplings. They took off in a really big way in the 1990s, spawning all kinds of variations – including *takoyaki*-flavoured crisps and pizza. As long as you can avoid thinking of testicles when biting through the crisp exterior into the soft, chewy interior, they are delicious. We include a recipe on page 53.

The truth is, however, that octopus doesn't deserve to be treated as a bizarre, unusual or macho ingredient suitable only for those with steely nerves, cast-iron stomachs, and non-squeamish dispositions. It's delicious, healthy, easy to cook, cheap and – crucially in this age of over-exploited fisheries – it can be sustainable.

A SUSTAINABLE SEAFOOD

Octopuses have many features that make for a highly sustainable resource. For example, the most important food species, O. vulgaris, has a short lifespan (one to five years), grows quickly, reaches sexual maturity early, and has high reproductive rates (females produce between 50,000 and 750,000 eggs). These features are broadly shared by other commercially important octopus species, making them particularly resistant to predation or fishing pressure.

There is also very little to waste. For a typical fish, the edible flesh is about 50 per cent of the total weight, and the actual yield (that is, skinless fillets) can be as low as half of that. This means that up to three-quarters of a fish may be discarded.

Not so the octopus. The edible portion of a typical octopus is about 90 per cent of its total weight, higher even than for squid. Actual commercial yields are not much lower, at around 80 per cent. (Octopuses are also themselves very efficient at turning food into body mass.)

Catching octopuses is relatively straightforward. They live in dens – essentially, any suitable hole where they can hide during the day or when not out hunting. They prefer to move to a new den every few days, so are always on the lookout for a suitable spot. Fishermen take advantage of this by placing enticing containers – traditionally, clay pots, now often PVC pipes – on the sea floor, and collecting them a day or so later to check for octopuses. It is not even necessary to use any bait. This time-honoured fishing method is highly selective – in the sense that only the targeted species is caught – and it does minimal damage to the marine environment. Unfortunately, fishing for octopus is not always carried out using sustainable techniques. While some fisheries, particularly those targeting high-value specimens in well-regulated inshore areas (such as Spain), use pot methods, many fisheries use bottom trawls (called 'otter trawls'), which are very destructive to the marine environment.

The North African octopus fishery has historically been the largest O. vulgaris fishery in the world. At its peak in 1994, it had a catch of 135,000 tons of octopus, according to the Food and Agriculture Organization of the United Nations. This is a trawl fishery that specifically targets octopus, mainly in the waters off Morocco and Mauritania (the latter being heavily overfished, with octopus stocks regarded as being in critical condition). Much of the catch is exported to Japan for processing, both for the local market and for re-export. Vietnam, Indonesia and the Philippines also have major octopus fisheries, their stocks are considered to be heavily exploited and management practices poor. In addition to its sustainable pot fishery, Spain also has a large trawl fishery, which is reasonably-well regulated; it mostly serves the domestic market. There are numerous other trawl fisheries around the world that catch significant quantities of octopus – sometimes as a target species, but in many cases as by-catch. Some of these trawl fisheries are managed better than others. (There are also, by the way, some non-targeted but highly sustainable octopus fisheries – for example, the octopuses caught in crab and lobster pots. In some cases, economic analyses have shown that the profits from catching octopus outweigh the losses from predation of the target species by those octopuses.)

Unfortunately for the consumer, there is often little reliable information on where the octopus they buy has been sourced. This means that while octopus has the potential to be a highly sustainable seafood, in practice this is not always the case. As always, get to know your fishmonger, and try to find out where the octopus you buy is sourced. The more popular octopus becomes, and the greater the demand for quality, the greater the economic incentive for producers to selectively fish them in a sustainable way. It is certainly no coincidence that the Spanish, who eat more octopus per capita than any other country, also have among the most sustainable octopus fisheries.

Octopus aquaculture

Aquaculture is big business, accounting for more than one-quarter of global seafood production. So it's not surprising that there has been considerable interest in farming octopus. They are particularly suited to aquaculture, being highly tolerant of captive conditions, having high reproductive and growth rates, a short life-cycle, and also because in some markets there is strong demand and high prices. So far, however, the few commercial ventures that exist (such as in Japan, South Korea and Spain) rely on raising wild-caught juveniles in sea cages. Successful raising of larval octopus on a commercial basis, and the development of appropriate artificial diets, will both be required before octopus aquaculture can take off. While there may be commercial justifications for such an approach, as with many other forms of aquaculture, the environmental benefits are less certain. Effective management of wild octopus populations must remain the priority.

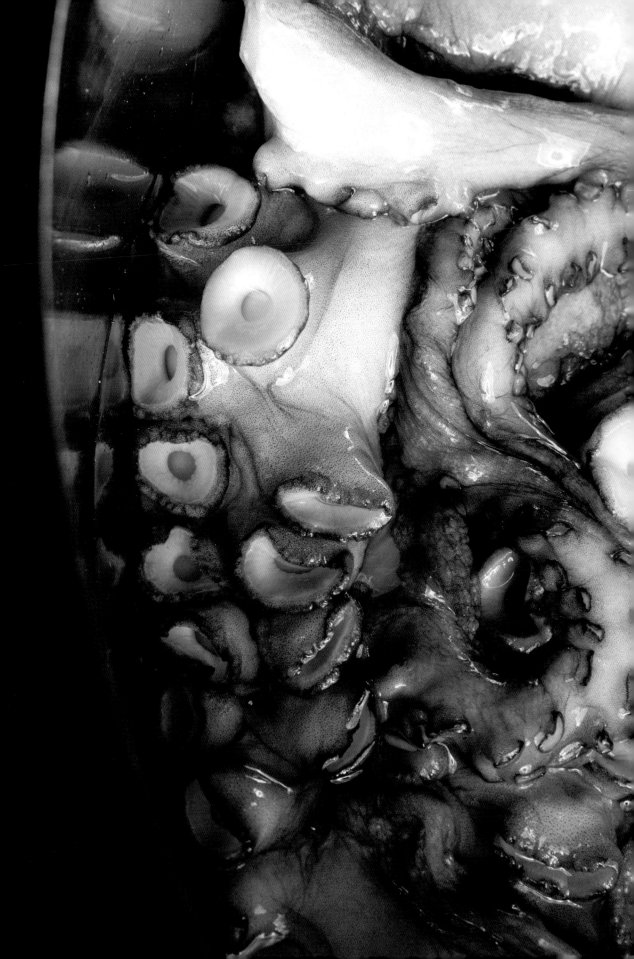

Eat me tender

THE FOUR BS

Octopus has a reputation for being tough. So much so, that almost every recipe you will find for octopus comes with strict instructions to follow some arcane tenderisation procedure, each more bizarre than the next. Failure to do so, the reader is warned, will turn the octopus into old boots. We have come across all of the following pronouncements in published recipes: the octopus must be beaten repeatedly on a rock; bashed with a mallet; churned in a cement mixer (preferably with some rocks thrown in); spun in a washing machine; hung overnight; frozen for a fortnight; or definitely not frozen; rubbed with grated daikon radish; or beaten repeatedly with whole peeled daikon; or massaged for an extended period (with or without salt); dipped exactly three times in boiling water before simmering; stored in seawater; brined; simmered with some vinegar; or tonic water; or with a wine cork; or with half a potato; or with dried soy beans; or wrapped in papaya leaves; or cooked only in a copper pan; or in any old pan with some copper coins thrown in. In *Toilers of the Sea*, Victor Hugo described (live) octopus arms as 'supple as leather, tough as steel, cold as night'. It hardly sounds like something you'd want to eat. Is octopus worth the bother?

We think this reputation for toughness is thoroughly undeserved, and that most of the proposed remedies are nonsense. It seems to us that they go hand-in-hand with the exoticism of the beast itself: octopuses are bizarre, mystical creatures; and they need to be cooked in bizarre, mystical ways. It's hard to imagine the same thing happening with the humble, familiar cow. Badly cooked or over-cooked steak can be tough as leather. But the remedy is simple: no bizarre rituals are necessary – you just learn to cook it properly. It's the same with octopus. You don't need a culinary High Priest to instruct you how to cook it, you just need some basic cooking technique.

And what of its texture? In part, it depends on which of the cooking methods described in this chapter you employ. Charlie Trotter says octopus has a 'slightly chewy eloquence'. That about sums up braised or boiled octopus for us – wonderfully tender with a slight chewy resistance. Blanched octopus has a very different texture. It's definitely less tender, but more crunchy than chewy. Some people might find it to be tough, but that's definitely no reason to eschew (if you'll excuse the term) blanching. We love it, and we suspect that many people who might complain about its toughness would happily chew away on a piece of over-cooked steak that we would consign to the bin. Similarly, dried octopus, while not as tender as octopus that has been braised or boiled, is definitely not tough.

To Clean an Octopus

Turn the mantle inside out and remove the innards. These pull away without too much effort, and you can cut any tough membranes. Among the innards is the ink sac – locate it and set aside if your recipe calls for it. Discard the rest. Next, remove the beak and its housing (the 'buccal mass'). This is located inside the mouth hole, at the centre point where the arms meet. It can be pushed out of the mouth hole by applying pressure from the other side. Next, cut off the eyes and discard. Rinse the octopus well under running water, and check there is no sand in the suckers (it can be removed by squeezing the sucker from the sides). Lastly, turn the mantle the right way round, so the octopus skin is on the outside.

As far as preparing your octopus before cooking is concerned, there is little – well, nothing – to do. They lack not only a back-bone, but in fact have no internal skeleton at all – not even the internal shells of their cousins the squid (which have a stiff 'pen') and cuttlefish (which have a 'bone'). Their beak is the only hard part of their body and that, along with the eyes, brain and other internal organs will have been removed from the head by your fishmonger. If for any reason these parts have not been removed, it's easy to do.

The four Bs represent our core techniques for octopus preparation. In the recipes that follow you can see the huge number of ways these techniques can be supplemented with others to make a range of delicious dishes.

Under Pressure

Not everyone likes pressure cookers. We're not sure why. They have a range of uses: cooking pulses and vegetables in double-quick time, tenderising tough cuts much more quickly than normal or even just cooking octopus. To be honest, we think the results of cooking octopus in a pressure cooker alone make it worth getting one. It simply is the easiest, best and most foolproof way we know to get tasty tender octopus every time.

Simply put one or more cleaned octopus in a pressure cooker – do not add any water. Bring up to full pressure for 15 minutes, then allow to cool a little. The result is beautifully tender and flavourful octopus. Enough juices are released that there's no risk of it sticking, and these juices produce a wonderful sauce, packed with octopus flavour, and faintly redolent of the sea. The gelatine from the skin gives it a great mouth-feel. You can reduce the sauce by half to thicken it and concentrate the flavours, then whisk in a little unsalted butter, and season with a few turns of white pepper. Pour this sauce over chunks of the cooked flesh, and you're in octopus heaven.

Braise

This is the easiest way – and we think by far the best way – to cook octopus. Braising in a pressure cooker produces consistently tender results. See below for how it's done.

If you don't have a pressure cooker, we'd recommend you get one. It's easier and much quicker, and because it's sealed to keep in the steam, the pressure cooker also locks in all the flavour. But you can reproduce similar results in the oven. Put the cleaned octopus in a heavy, ovenproof pan with a lid, and cook in a 90°C oven until tender, about 4-5 hours. Allow the octopus to cool a little in its juices, remove from the pan, then reduce the liquid as above. Make sure that the pan you use is not too big for the quantity of octopus, or there's a risk that the juices may burn off rather than providing a braising liquid for the flesh. As long as the octopus covers at least two-thirds of the base of the pan, you should be ok. See the box below for how to cook sous vide – a high tech version of braising that is very effective.

Braising, high-tech style

A high-tech alternative to braising is 'sous vide'. Initially the preserve of top-end restaurant kitchens using expensive equipment from laboratory suppliers to prepare everything from foie gras to fish and fruit, in recent years it has become more accessible to the home cook and we think in the future sous vide will be as mainstream as the microwave.

The technique allows for very accurate control of cooking temperature, which means reliable and repeatable results. The food to be cooked is vacuum sealed in plastic pouches, then cooked in a water bath kept at a constant (and often fairly low) temperature. This has enabled chefs to produce such wonders as beef short ribs that have been cooked for 72 hours until meltingly tender, but are still rare because of the low cooking temperature. Ideally, you need a chamber vacuum sealer to seal the food before cooking, but these are very expensive; however, it's possible to achieve good results with a domestic 'food saver'-type sealer – in fact, even a zip-loc bag can work. The cooking process requires an immersion circulator (a device that heats water to a specific temperature, and circulates it to keep that temperature constant). Several options are now available for the home cook, including the excellent 'Joule' from Chef Steps (a UK version is expected soon) and a similar device from Anova. If you want to try this technique, we recommend that you get to grips with the basics by reading one of the books or internet sites dedicated to it – chefsteps.com is a great place to start.

For a high-tech braise, seal cleaned octopus in a bag with a herb sachet (a bay leaf and some peppercorns, loosely wrapped in a small piece of cling film so that the flavours can get out, but the herbs don't come into direct contact with the octopus) and cook for 4 hours at 82°C. The results will be well worth it: firm but tender octopus, with a delicate flavour, and lovely pink juices for a sauce. After removing the octopus from the bag, we like to sear it briefly on a hot griddle for added flavour.

Braising in one of these ways produces such fantastic results that this could be the only octopus-cooking technique you ever need. You should never end up with tough or rubbery results, and the taste will be incomparable – it will taste of octopus, a subtle, wonderful flavour that most other cooking techniques end up masking, rather than enhancing. And if you do want to introduce different flavours, you can do that too. Try adding a chopped onion (raw, or browned in a little butter or olive oil) and a bouquet garni with the octopus, and perhaps a dash of red wine vinegar to the sauce after you've reduced it, to cut through the richness. Add some chopped parsley to the sauce just before serving, or infuse a bunch of parsley in the reduced sauce for a few minutes, then remove before whisking in the butter.

You can reflect whatever recipe your octopus is going to be used for by introducing different ingredients into the braise. So for a Mediterranean touch try some oregano, tarragon or saffron; for a more Southeast Asian flavour add ginger, garlic and chilli, or even lemongrass. Use your imagination – but respect the THE MAXIM OF PURITY.

Boil

Another great technique for octopus is to cook it slowly in a flavoured liquid (a court-bouillon, or 'nage'). Although we refer to it as 'boiling', the idea is to keep the liquid at a slow simmer, rather than a rapid boil. Cooked for the right amount of time – until the point of a knife will easily penetrate the thickest part of an arm – and the result is reliably tender, flavourful octopus that can be used as it is, or as a basis for fried or grilled octopus dishes.

A classic court bouillon is made with onion, leek, celery, carrot and garlic, together with a bouquet garni. But as with braising, it's easy to infuse the octopus with different flavours, by adding different ingredients to the cooking liquid – or by replacing the court bouillon with red or white wine.

Blanch

Braising and boiling both produce tender, lobster-like octopus by cooking it long enough that the tough connective tissue breaks down (even if that happens pretty quickly in a pressure cooker). Blanching, however, avoids toughness by very quick cooking, so that the muscle fibres do not have a chance to contract enough to toughen the flesh. The result is a completely different – almost crunchy – texture that, while it may not be to everyone's liking, is certainly not tough. We love it cooked this way in certain dishes (such as the Hawaiian Poke on page 38); but this is definitely an alternative method, rather than a mainstay.

It's really very simple. Bring a pot of water, deep enough to completely cover the octopus, to a rolling boil. Submerge the cleaned octopus in the boiling water for 2–3 minutes, depending on the size of your beast. Then remove and refresh immediately in a large bowl of ice water. (The aim is to chill the octopus very quickly, to stop the cooking process, so plenty of ice is required.) Once the octopus is thoroughly cooled, it's ready to be incorporated into your recipe.

Brine?

Well, not quite. While we're both big fans of brining meat, we don't think that brining octopus produces great results. We've experimented a lot with this, and while it's clear that brining has a major effect, we find that the technique spoils both the texture and the flavour. In short, given that the other methods discussed above produce fantastic, tender results, there's no reason to brine octopus.

Dry

No, our fourth and final 'B' actually begins with a 'D'. But hey, only one of the educational three 'R's (reading, writing and 'rithmetic) begins with an 'R'. We love to dry octopus, and find that it has a great effect on the texture and the flavour. As with other foods that are 'dried', a great deal depends on the degree of drying that actually takes place: in physiological terms, just how much water is driven out of the octopus itself. In order to preserve octopus by drying (or – for that matter – any foodstuff), the general rule is that the water content of the food in question should be reduced to 15 per cent or less. At this rate of desiccation, not only has all the bacterial activity that spoils the food been arrested, but moulds also cannot grow. If you live in a warm, dry climate, and you have a glut of octopus, this may be a method you would like to explore. Simply lay it out on racks in the sun until it feels completely dry. The smell and taste of the octopus will be heightened, and you can either choose to reconstitute it at your leisure, by soaking it in water – in which case treat the octopus as fresh and either braise or blanch – or follow the lead of the late George Lassalle. Lassalle was a visionary cookery writer, and he describes in his book *The Adventurous Fish Cook* the way he enjoyed dried octopus bought in London's Chinatown before World War II:

> These withered objects were exciting to cook... They should be thrown on to a very hot griddle, when the performance will begin. For a short time, nothing seems likely to happen; then, suddenly, movement will be detected and the beast will start to come alive, gently writhing and stretching its eight tentacles in an attempt to sing as they touch the hot plate. When one side is cooked almost to singeing and has turned a blackish purple, it should be turned over and again cooked to singeing.

For most of us, drying octopus to this extent is impractical. But there is more to drying than just preserving, and there are other reasons to dry. The flavour of fresh tomatoes is greatly enhanced by halving them and placing them in a slow oven (70°C) for 4–5 hours. Essentially, what this process does is replicate the effect of being slow-cooked by the sun. The tomatoes will emerge from the oven with their water content reduced and their natural sugars concentrated. They will be so sweet. So it is with octopus. Almost all of the grilled octopus you eat in restaurants in Greece will have been 'half'-dried in a similar way. The octopus is simply hung outside in the warm breeze for 24 hours (we have learned the hard way that it must be out of reach of local felines). In the semi-dry state that results, it can be grilled over charcoal (no need to boil or blanch first), then sprinkled with a little salt, some olive oil and lemon, and the result is marvellous. As with octopus that has been blanched, it is not quite as tender as that which has been braised (either in a pressure cooker or oven), but it is certainly not tough.

Armed with the four Bs (well, 3 Bs and a D) you need never fear cooking octopus. In the next chapter we provide a range of delicious recipes: some straightforward, others more challenging. Most recipes call for Braising or Boiling, and you can in many cases use either method. Some recipes specify Blanching, when we think that the alternative, slightly crunchy octopus texture we describe above works better. (Blanching can also be done very quickly, and sometimes we just can't wait to sit down to a light octopus supper). However, if you prefer your octopus tender, yet with that chewy eloquence, by all means braise or boil instead of blanching for these recipes. The final, short section contains a number of ways of using either semi-dried or completely dried octopus.

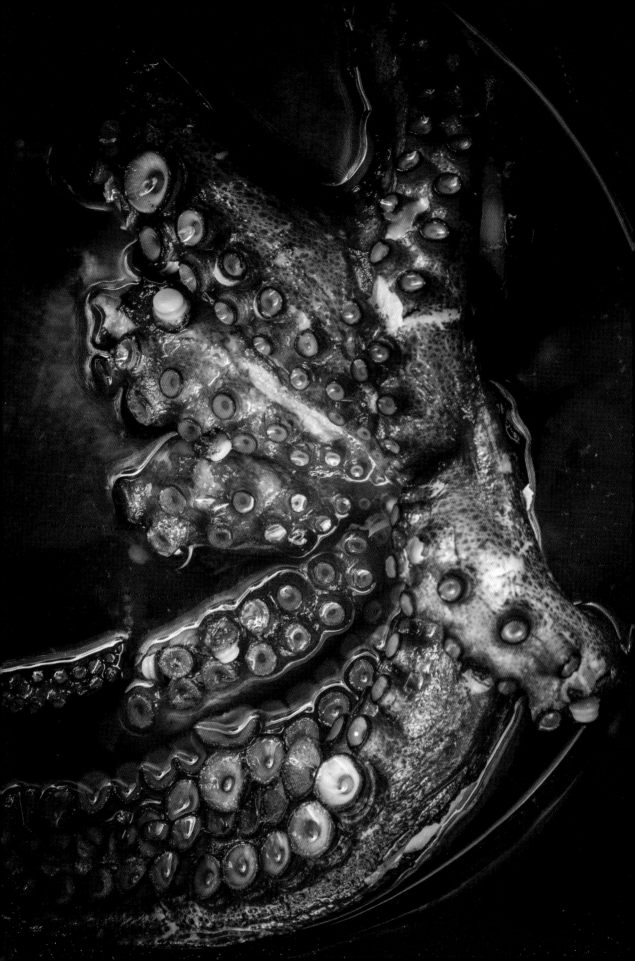

RECIPES

All recipes serve 4 unless otherwise noted.

COOL AND REFRESHING

A whole constellation of delicious, refreshing, healthy dishes cluster around the generic term 'salad': but what is a salad? One clue is that the word 'salad' is nearly the same in all European languages, deriving as it does from the Latin word for salt – 'sal'. So we have the French 'salade', Italian 'insalada', Spanish 'ensalada', German 'salat', Swedish 'sallad' and so on. Salt, then, is crucial (we'll leave it up to you to decide whether fruit salads are 'salads'). Of course, in Oriental and Pacific cuisine the salty note is often provided by an Asian fish sauce – 'nam pla' – just as in Roman times it was provided by 'garum', the entrails of salted fish fermented in barrels. But it is salt just the same.

Other essential seasonings in a salad include an acidic element – usually vinegar or lemon juice (though we find white wine sometimes makes an agreeable change) and an oil. This might be a neutral oil such as vegetable, sunflower or peanut, or a rich flavoursome one such as extra virgin olive oil, hazelnut oil or walnut oil.

Salads themselves generally fall into a number of distinct classes: salads made of just leaves ('green' salads), salads made of vegetables (potato salad, roasted bell pepper salad, 'Russian' salad), poultry or fowl salads, meat salads and fish or seafood salads. We find, needless to say, that an octopus salad is among the very best of all salads.

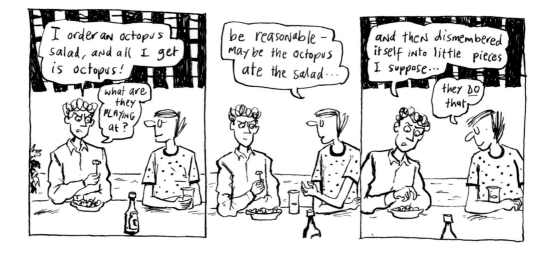

Vietnamese Octopus Salad

This recipe is adapted from one by Australian chefs Luke Nguyen and Mark Jensen. Luke Nguyen is now something of a fixture on British television cooking channels – his enthusiasm for Vietnamese food and culture is infectious and he's a great communicator.

1 medium octopus (about 500g cleaned weight)

60ml Asian fish sauce

30ml lemon juice

10g palm sugar (or brown sugar)

2 cloves garlic, finely chopped

1 tablespoon vegetable oil

300g cucumber, peeled and deseeded and cut into thin strips

80g red onion, cut into thin slices

10 cherry tomatoes, halved

1 lemongrass stalk, outer leaves removed, finely sliced

a few sprigs of purple-stemmed basil (*húng quế* or Thai basil), cut into chiffonade

1 teaspoon toasted rice powder

1 tablespoon chopped roasted peanuts

1 hot red chilli, seeds and pith removed and finely sliced

salt and rice vinegar

1. Blanch the octopus (see page 32). Set aside to cool.

2. Combine the fish sauce, lemon juice, sugar, garlic and oil in a bowl and mix well. Add the cooled octopus and leave to marinate for 30 minutes to an hour.

3. Meanwhile, combine the cucumber, onion, tomatoes, lemongrass and basil in a bowl. Add the toasted rice powder (you can easily make this yourself by toasting a little jasmine rice in a dry pan until light brown, then grinding once it has cooled).

4. Drain the octopus, reserving the marinade. Grill or barbecue over high heat for a few minutes on each side until lightly charred. Cut into bite-sized pieces and add to the salad.

5. Adjust the seasoning of the reserved marinade, adding salt and rice vinegar to taste. Add 2 to 3 tablespoons to the salad and mix well. Serve garnished with the peanuts and red chilli.

Octopus Ceviche, Peruvian style

Ceviche is a classic of South and Central American cuisine. Normally, raw fish or shellfish is used, with the acidic marinade (citrus juice or vinegar) causing the proteins to denature, similar to the effect of the cooking process. When octopus is used, however, it is generally cooked first. In Peru, the very hot and aromatic *ají* chilli is traditionally used in ceviche.

1 medium-large octopus (800g – 1 kg cleaned weight)
400g sweet potatoes, boiled, peeled and sliced thinly
court bouillon
200g tomatoes, peeled, seeded and diced
2 jalapeno chillies (or other hot chilli),
seeds and pith removed and chopped fine
100g red onion, cut into thin strips
50ml lime juice (and zest for garnish)
2 tablespoons chopped coriander leaves (and more for garnish)
30ml olive oil
salt and freshly-ground black pepper

1. Boil the sweet potato, drain, and leave to cool.

2. Meanwhile, boil the cleaned octopus in a court bouillon (see page 32). Reserve 2 tablespoons of the cooking liquid. When the octopus has cooled, cut off the head and set aside for another purpose. Slice the arms into bite-sized pieces.

3. Mix the octopus pieces together with the tomatoes, chillies and onion.

4. Whisk together the reserved octopus cooking liquid (which should be cool), lime juice and coriander. Add to the octopus mix and toss well. Allow to marinate for a few minutes (and up to a day, in the fridge). Add the olive oil and mix well. Adjust the seasoning. Garnish with a little lime zest and a sprig of coriander. Serve at room temperature with slices of boiled sweet potato.

Hawaiian Octopus Poke

Poke (pronounced 'po-kay') is a Hawaiian word meaning 'to cut', and it is the name given to a traditional Hawaiian dish, typically served as a snack or appetiser. At its most basic, poke consists of cubes of raw seafood mixed with seaweed and a relish made of the local kukui nut ('candlenut'). But there are many variations, and it has become something of a national dish, with Hawaiian chefs competing to out-do each other at an annual poke contest. As with other dishes based on raw seafood (such as sushi or ceviche), when octopus is used it is normally cooked – raw, it has little flavour and the consistency of elastic.

Here are two recipes, a very traditional one using ingredients that might be hard to come by outside of Hawaii, and our own non-traditional interpretation.

Traditional:

1 medium octopus (about 500g cleaned weight)
50g finely chopped yellow onion
50g finely chopped spring onion
30g *limu kohu* (a red seaweed similar to the Irish dulse)
10g *inamona* (a paste made from ground roasted kukui nut kernels)
10ml sesame oil
sea salt

1. Blanch the cleaned octopus (see page 32), plunge into an ice-bath, then cut into small pieces. Mix together with all the other ingredients.

2. Serve at room temperature.

It is possible to substitute a couple of crushed Japanese nori sheets for the red seaweed. There are no real substitutes for the kukui nuts/*inamona* – some people suggest using crushed roasted macadamia nuts, but although these have a similar consistency, the taste is very different.

Our version:

1 medium octopus (about 500g cleaned weight)
1 hot red chilli, seeds and pith removed, finely chopped
5ml sesame oil
5ml dark soy sauce
juice and finely-grated zest of a lime
half a teaspoon of finely grated ginger
1 ripe medium-sized tomato, chopped
half a cucumber, peeled and diced
1 spring onion, white and pale green parts only, thinly sliced
sea salt

1. Blanch the cleaned octopus, plunge into an ice-bath, then cut into small pieces.

2. Mix together the chilli, oil, soy, lime zest and juice, ginger, then toss with the tomato, cucumber, spring onion and octopus.

3. Add salt to taste. Serve at room temperature.

Portuguese Octopus Salad (Sr Rocha's Salata do Polvo)

The Portuguese have some wonderful ways with octopus. Indeed, all over the Iberian Peninsula the ingredient is treated with great reverence. In Galicia, the westernmost province of continental Europe, the locals hold an annual 'Festa do Polbo' in which hundreds of kilos of octopuses are boiled up and served on small wooden platters as Polbo a Feira. Indeed, the Spanish term for octopus salad is Pulpo a la Gallega (Octopus the Galician way): cubes of octopus sprinkled with paprika, each cube impaled on a cocktail stick on one of those familiar wooden platters make a very popular tapas dish.

The gentleman who provided this recipe – Sr Armando Rocha, of Penafirme, Torres Vedras – would have had little doubt, however, that it is the Portuguese version of this salad that is the original.

As with many salads, this recipe is more about assembly than it is about cooking. The most important thing is that both the octopus and the potatoes are warm while the salad is being prepared. This way, the oil seems to marry with the octopus and potatoes in a way that simply doesn't happen when the ingredients are cold. (The same is true of a plain potato salad.)

1 medium-large octopus (800g – 1 kg cleaned weight)
4 or 5 boiled potatoes in their skins
2 onions, chopped
2 cloves garlic, chopped
small bunch parsley or coriander, chopped
200ml extra virgin olive oil
salt and freshly-ground black pepper

1. Braise or boil the octopus.

2. Cut the octopus arms into one or two pieces each and slice the mantle thinly.

3. Skin the potatoes and cut them into pieces (be careful to make sure that the pieces are not too small – a potato the size of a medium apple should yield four to five pieces).

4. Arrange both the warm octopus and the potato pieces on a serving dish.

5. Strew with chopped onion (again, not chopped too small) and garlic.

6. Season well with sea salt and sprinkle with chopped parsley or coriander and lots of oil.

7. Serve with crusty bread, and more olive oil.

There is something deeply comforting about the combination of the tender octopus pieces, the earthy potatoes, the crisp cool onion and fruity olive oil. Salads such as these exist all over southern continental Europe but are spurned in the north. As we saw a few years ago, in Germany – for example – an octopus has more chance of a career in football punditry than making it to the pot.

At Christmas time in mid-Portugal, when a salad is the last thing on your mind, families adapt the above recipe. Firstly, it is covered with cooked as opposed to raw onions, then strewn with slices of spicy Portuguese sausage (*chouriço*) together with red chillies. It is then baked in a medium oven for 45 minutes or so. The potatoes roast to a crisp deliciousness, and the octopus becomes darker, more meaty and even more intensely flavoured. Prepared in this way you have Polvo Assado no Forno: give us this over roast turkey any day.

On Salt

You'll notice we recommend that you season this dish 'well'. We don't necessarily mean that you should add a huge amount of salt to your food, but at the very least we think it's worth seasoning food, tasting it and (if necessary) seasoning it again. The Salt Police are everywhere and we know many people who proudly claim never to add salt to their food. But unseasoned food lacks flavour. And people who don't add salt often eat processed food that contains far higher salt levels (often masked with other ingredients) than a properly seasoned meal cooked at home with fresh ingredients. The health risks of salt are often over-stated: people who already have high blood pressure may benefit from reducing their salt intake, but there is much less evidence that a low-salt diet is beneficial for people with normal blood pressure, or that it prevents the development of high blood pressure. Japan, a country whose per capita salt consumption is greater than anywhere in Europe or the US, has one of the highest life expectancies in the world. The truth is that the best thing we can do for our dietary heath is eat a balance of fresh, nutritious – and yes, flavourful – foods.

Greek Octopus Salad (Octapodhiasalata)

On the face of it, the Greek version of octopus salad is very similar to those enjoyed by the Portuguese and Spanish. However, it differs in two crucial ways, which makes the Greek octopus salad an entirely different kettle of cephalopod. Firstly, before being cooked the octopus is half-dried in the sun as described in the previous section. If you are fortunate to be based – either permanently or temporarily – in a part of the world where this is feasible, then you simply must try it: the flavour is concentrated so much, and the texture beautiful in the mouth. Secondly, rather than being braised or boiled beforehand, the octopus arms are put directly onto the bars of a charcoal grill and left to cook slowly until they are cooked through and slightly charred. The arms are then cut into very thin rounds (which means that one octopus goes a long way). Eleni and Lefteris Niniou of the Big Blue Taverna, Vathi, Sifnos cut theirs into rounds no thicker than a coin. Served with lots of olive oil and a small amount of lemon juice or red wine vinegar, this is sensational with a glass of ouzo or a cold beer. Indeed, in parts of Greece that have resisted the rise of tourism, a small portion of octopus cooked in this way is an obligatory – and complimentary – accompaniment to a glass of ouzo.

Italian Salad of Octopus, Rocket and Apples
(Insalata di Polpo e Rucola)

This is an adaptation of a recipe provided in the seminal Italian cookery book *Il Cucchiaio d'Argento* ('The Silver Spoon').

The size of the octopus pieces is quite important here, since the objective is that in each mouthful you will have octopus, rocket, pine nut and apple. We have made the recipe successfully with watercress instead of rocket.

1 medium octopus (about 500g cleaned weight)
a large bunch of rocket
3 tablespoons of pine nuts
half an apple, cored and diced quite finely
100ml extra virgin olive oil
juice of half a lemon, strained
salt and freshly-ground black pepper

1. Braise or boil the octopus.

2. Tear the rocket leaves in two if they are large and mix with the pine nuts and diced apple.

3. Slice the octopus arms and mantle into quite small pieces (not as small as for a Greek octopus salad, but smaller than for Portuguese).

4. Mix the octopus with the rocket, pine nut and apple mixture.

5. Whisk the olive oil and lemon juice together and season with salt and pepper.

6. Toss the whole mixture together and serve.

HOT AND WARMING

Octopus is a highly versatile ingredient and is as much at home in a salad as it is in some of the hot, warming dishes we provide below.

Spicy North African Octopus Soup

Variations of this spicy soup are popular in Tunisia, Algeria and other parts of north Africa.

1 medium-large octopus (800g – 1kg cleaned weight)

50ml olive oil

1 medium onion, finely chopped

1 medium carrot, finely chopped

1 stick of celery, finely chopped

3 cloves of garlic, finely chopped

4 dried red chillies, broken into pieces

500g tomatoes, peeled, seeded and chopped

1 tablespoon caraway seeds

1 teaspoon cumin seeds

1 tablespoon coriander seeds

1 teaspoon cayenne powder

100g bulgur wheat (coarse), rinsed

20g coriander leaves, whole with stems removed

2 lemons

salt and freshly-ground black pepper

1. Blanch the octopus, then cut into bite-sized pieces and reserve.

2. Heat the oil in a large heavy-bottomed pan over medium heat. Sauté the onion, carrot and celery, stirring occasionally, until the onion is soft (about 20

minutes). Add the garlic, chilli and some salt and black pepper and sauté for a further 2 minutes.

3. Add the tomatoes and simmer, stirring, until most of the liquid has evaporated, about 15–20 minutes.

4. Meanwhile, toast the caraway, cumin and coriander seeds in a dry pan until fragrant. Allow to cool, then break up in a pestle and mortar (or grind briefly in a spice grinder/ blender). Add to the tomatoes along with the cayenne.

5. When the tomatoes are ready, add the pieces of octopus and 2 litres of water. Simmer for at least an hour, until the octopus is tender. Add the bulgur and 15g of the coriander leaves in the last 20 minutes of cooking, reserving the remaining coriander leaves for garnish.

6. When cooked, adjust seasoning and add lemon juice to taste. Serve, garnished with coriander leaves, and lemon wedges on the side.

Portuguese Octopus Rice (Arroz do Polvo)

About fifty metres away from Armando Rocha's house was, and perhaps still is, a large seaside restaurant offering a range of Portuguese dishes: you could drop in for a cheap snack – a custard tart, a sandwich or a plate of small salt cod fritters – or choose from a selection of freshly-caught fish or shellfish. In the early 90s it was possible for two people to eat (and drink) like royalty and emerge having spent about 1500 escudos (around £5). The Portuguese have evolved their own unique rice dishes flavoured with tomato, red pepper, garlic, coriander and chilli and these dishes were the speciality of this restaurant. They are cooked and served in earthenware dishes of various sizes and contain rice and a range of delicious seafood. As well as Arroz do Polvo, other notable dishes include Arroz do Tamboril (anglerfish rice) and Arroz do Mariscos (mixed shellfish rice).

We have not experienced rice dishes anything like them anywhere else on our travels. Like the Italian risotto, the rice is not expected to emerge dry – as it is in many Eastern rice dishes – but instead coated with the stock in which it has been cooked. Unlike risotto, however, broth and liquid do not marry together into a homogenous, creamy mass. Rather, the final dish appears as liquid as a soup when it first appears at the table, with the rice and main ingredients (octopus, or anglerfish, or lobster) invisible beneath (in other words much more liquid than an authentic Italian risotto). As well as this, and again unlike risotto and paella, long-grained rice is used.

1 medium-large octopus (800g – 1kg cleaned weight)

50ml olive oil

1 red pepper, sliced a few cloves of garlic, chopped
1 onion, sliced
200ml of tomato passata
(or some fresh tomatoes, peeled, deseeded and cooked down to a pulp)
250g long grain rice
2 bay leaves
salt, freshly-ground black pepper, lemon juice

1. Braise or boil the octopus, making sure you reserve either the liquid that emerges during braising, or the water in which the octopus has been boiled. Cut into bite-sized pieces and reserve.

2. Pour the oil into a large pan and cook the red pepper, garlic and onion until they are all softened. Add the tomato passata and reduce by about half.

3. Add the octopus liquor. You'll need about 500ml. If you have braised your octopus, simply dilute the concentrated octopus liquor with enough water to give you the required amount. If you've boiled it, then strain the cooking liquid and reduce if necessary to 500ml.

4. Once the liquor is boiling, add the octopus, rice, bay leaves and seasonings.

5. Simmer for about 20 minutes until the rice is cooked.

6. Season with salt, pepper and lemon juice, strew chopped coriander over the whole and serve.

For an authentic Arroz do Polvo, remember that the whole thing should be quite liquid when served. You may need to add more liquid if the rice has absorbed most of the liquor you added at the beginning. If this is the case, remember to taste for seasoning. It's not strictly authentic, but we often season our (fishy) rice dishes with *nam pla* rather than salt. It helps add to the depth of flavour. Note also that not all Arroz do Polvo recipes include red pepper. The dish served in this restaurant, however, certainly did, and a most welcome addition it was.

Risotto Nero with Octopus

This dish is a variation on the famous Risotto Nero (black rice) of Venice. The risotto traditionally contains cuttlefish, and is flavoured and coloured with cuttlefish ink. The octopus, of course, is also a prodigious ink-producer and we think this is just as good as the original.

1 medium-large octopus (800g – 1kg cleaned weight) including ink sac

50ml olive oil

1 onion, sliced

250g Arborio (or Carnaroli) rice

100ml white wine

parsley

1. Braise or boil the octopus, making sure you reserve either the liquid that emerges during braising, or the water in which the octopus has been boiled. To this you add the octopus ink. This will give you a very black stock, which you must keep bubbling away while you prepare the onion. (If you have only the braising liquid, you'll need to add water. You'll need about 650ml of stock in total.)

2. Pour the oil into a large pan and cook the onion until softened.

3. Add the rice and stir gently until it is amalgamated with the onion and each grain is glistening with oil.

4. Add the wine and reduce until almost evaporated.

5. Add a ladleful of octopus liquor to the rice and keep stirring until it too has almost evaporated.

6. Repeat stage 5 until the rice is nicely al dente.

7. Add the octopus pieces to your risotto, cover with a lid and leave to rest for 3 minutes or so and then serve with sprinkling of parsley. Strictly no parmesan!

This dish is extraordinarily beautiful, the pale pieces of octopus arm flecked with purple, nestling in plump jet-black grains of rice.

Octopus Daube (Poulpe en daube)

The 'daube' is one of those legendary dishes of Provence in southern France: a slow cooked casserole or stew of beef, red wine, vegetables and spices. Even cooked in a domestic oven, the smell that emerges from a *daube* is amazing. What it must have smelt like being cooked over an open fire of vine cuttings and olive wood we can only imagine. In her classic book *French Provincial Cooking* Elizabeth David quotes a French cookery writer Pierre Huguenin describing it as follows:

> O, scent of the *daubes* of my childhood! During the holidays, at Gemeaux, in the month of August, when we arrived in my grandmother's dark kitchen on Sunday after Vespers, it was lit by a ray of sunshine in which the dust and the flies were dancing, and there was a sound like a little bubbling spring. It was a *daube*, which

since midday had been murmuring gently on the stove, giving out sweet smells which brought tears to your eyes. Thyme, rosemary, bay leaves, spices, the wine of the marinade and the *fumet* of the meat were becoming transformed under the magic wand which is the fire, into a delicious whole, which was served about seven o'clock in the evening, so well cooked and tender that it was carved with a spoon.

The meat of the octopus lends itself beautifully to the rich flavours of a *daube*. The following recipe is a version of one taken from J. B. Reboul's classic work on the cooking of the South of France, *La Cuisinière Provençale*. Notice that in Reboul's recipe the boiling of the octopus takes place with all the other ingredients, rather than beforehand. You could cook this recipe more quickly in a pressure cooker, but it would be a shame to deprive your loved ones of the aromas Huguenin describes.

1 medium-large octopus (800g–1kg cleaned weight)

1 bay leaf

thyme sprigs

sprig of flat-leaf parsley

150ml cognac

200g lardons of pork (unsmoked) – you could use olive oil instead

1 onion, chopped

2 tomatoes, chopped

3-4 cloves of garlic

200ml red or white wine (Reboul specifies white)

salt and freshly-ground black pepper

1. Cut the uncooked octopus into chunks and place them in a pan with salt, pepper, a bay leaf, a few sprigs of thyme and parsley and the cognac. Sauté the pieces until the liquid that emerges from the octopus has disappeared and the cognac has all but boiled away. Leave for a few hours.

2. Cook the lardons in a pot large enough to take all the ingredients until the fat is running well. Add the octopus (and all the aromatics) and the chopped onion, the tomatoes and the garlic. Let the onions soften and tomatoes boil down.

3. Add the white wine and the same quantity of water.

4. Put in a low oven and cook (the liquid should sound like a bubbling spring) until the octopus is very tender.

In Reboul's words: 'Le temps de cuisson reste subordonné a l'âge de bête' ('the cooking time depends on the age of the beast'). Reboul claims that an 'old' octopus will need 5–6 hours, a younger one between 2–3 hours. It is certainly true that large octopuses take longer to cook than smaller ones, but given the number of different species, size is not always an accurate indicator of age. Richard Olney suggests serving this with bread dried in the oven and spread with aioli, the garlic mayonnaise of the South of France. The combination is so utterly delicious that we include a recipe for aioli below. Please try it. Please.

Reboul's recipe is very similar to 'Kyria Eftychia's Octopus Stew' as provided in George Lassalle's *The Adventurous Fish Cook*, although she specifies red wine, some anchovy fillets and greater quantities of garlic. While Mrs Eftychia's version does not call for it, in Greece we have noticed that a small stick of cinnamon is an excellent addition to all Greek stews which use red wine (though if you add cinnamon, the aioli combination doesn't work so well).

Making Mayonnaise

The mystique surrounding the preparation of mayonnaise is completely overblown. We love making it, and if it really were the complex, drop-by-tiny-drop procedure it's sometimes described as, we'd never bother. The main thing to remember is this: the egg yolks should be at room temperature. If they're not, they will be stickier and it will be more difficult to get them to coat the droplets of oil, which is the essential part of the emulsification process. If the yolks are at room temperature, and are well whisked with a little mustard or vinegar, salt, and a little warm water too, the 'magical' emulsification process happens in a most reliable and un-magical way. A stick blender is good for incorporating the oil into the mixture, and while it's true that you need to add the oil slowly at the start, once the emulsion has formed you can add the rest with moderate abandon.

Aioli

Making your own mayonnaise is way easier than you think, see above.

several cloves of garlic (the more the better)

salt

2 egg yolks

some mustard powder (optional)

up to 500ml extra virgin olive oil

a squeeze of lemon

1. Pound the garlic to a paste with some salt in a pestle and mortar.

2. Mix in the egg yolks and a little salt, and mustard powder if using.

3. Begin incorporating the olive oil, slowly at first, then in a steady stream as the emulsion thickens.

4. By the time all the oil has been added the aioli will be a solid mass with a lovely oily lustre.

5. Check for salt.

6. If (like us) you are addicted to the stuff, you could add some aioli to the daube before you serve it.

Maldivian Curried Octopus (Miruhulee Boava)

Maldivian cuisine is heavily influenced by the cuisine of of Sri Lanka and southern India. And given that the Maldives is an archipelago of over 1,100 coral islands, seafood is ubiquitous. This spicy, fragrant octopus curry is a local favourite.

1 medium octopus (about 500g cleaned weight)

60ml coconut oil, ghee or butter

1 medium onion, finely chopped

10 cloves of garlic, finely chopped

2 teaspoons roughly chopped curry leaves

2 pandanus leaves (available fresh and dried from Asian shops)

3 teaspoons hot chilli flakes
(or several whole dried chillies; may be adjusted according to taste)

1 teaspoons cumin seeds

2 teaspoons black peppercorns

sea salt

1. Heat the oil and fry the onion and half the garlic together with the curry leaves and pandanus leaves, until the onion is lightly caramelised.

2. Meanwhile, make a paste from the remaining garlic, chilli, cumin and peppercorns, using a pestle and mortar (or a spice grinder/blender). Remove the arms from the octopus and cut into bite-sized pieces. (Reserve the mantle for another use.)

3. Once the onions are ready, add the octopus pieces and the spice paste, and season lightly with salt. Braise over a low heat until the octopus is tender, about 20 minutes.

4. Adjust seasoning and serve with steamed rice.

Octopus Gumbo

This is our alternative take on that Louisiana classic, which we think works wonderfully. The recipe is quite involved, but is worth it. You can make most of the recipe in advance. You can add more cayenne or some hot sauce for a more fiery version.

Prawn heads and shells make fantastic stock, and it's a pity to waste them. If you've got the time, make a stock from the heads and shells, then proceed with the rest of the recipe. Add the prawn stock together with the chicken stock. (To make a prawn stock, sauté the heads and shells in a little oil for a few minutes until crisp and bright, add water to cover, simmer for about 45 minutes, then strain.) If you don't have the time for this extra stage, freeze the heads and shells and make a stock at your leisure.

1 medium-large octopus (800g–1kg cleaned weight)

60g lard (or butter)

250g okra, cut crossways into 1cm slices, stalks removed

200g chorizo (or other spicy sausage), cut into 1cm slices

2 medium onions, finely diced

1 red bell pepper, seeded and finely diced

2 celery stalks, finely diced

4 garlic cloves, finely chopped

1 tablespoon chopped thyme leaves

25g (4 tablespoons) plain flour

600ml chicken stock (preferably home made)

125ml dry white wine

300g fresh tomatoes, peeled and chopped

1 bay leaf

1 teaspoon cayenne powder

400g medium-sized prawns

a little freshly squeezed lemon juice

chopped fresh flat-leaf parsley

salt and freshly-ground black pepper

1. Heat two teaspoons of the lard in a frying pan over medium heat. Add the okra and chorizo and sauté for a few minutes until the okra is lightly browned, being careful that it doesn't burn. Remove from the pan and set aside.

2. Return the frying pan to the heat. Add another two teaspoons of the lard. When hot, add the onions, pepper and celery and sauté, stirring occasionally, until the onion is soft (about 20 minutes). Add the garlic, thyme and some salt and black pepper and sauté for a further 2 minutes.

3. Meanwhile, make a dark roux as follows. Place a large heavy pot over medium-low heat. Add the rest of the fat, then when it is hot, stir in the flour. Continue stirring constantly until the mixture is a dark reddish-brown, about 15 minutes. Take care not to burn.

4. Gradually incorporate the chicken stock into the roux, stirring until smooth. Then add the wine, tomatoes, bay leaf, cayenne, sautéed vegetables, sautéed okra and chorizo. Simmer over low heat for about 40 minutes. You can make the gumbo in advance up to this point, and then store it in the fridge for up to three days. If anything, this improves the flavour.

5. On the day of service, braise the octopus (see p. 31). When cool enough to handle, cut into bite-sized pieces. Reserve the octopus juices. Peel and de-vein the prawns.

6. Bring the chilled gumbo sauce to a simmer, add the octopus and its juices, and bring back to a simmer. Add the prawns, and continue simmering until they are just cooked through, about 5 minutes.

7. Adjust seasoning and add a little lemon juice to taste, to cut through the richness. Garnish with chopped parsley and serve with steamed rice.

Tunisian Octopus with Cumin (Poulpe au Cumin)

This recipe is adapted from Alan Davidson's *Mediterranean Seafood*. His recipe calls for *octopus macropus* (the 'white-spotted' octopus), but it is so delicious it seems a shame not to cook other kinds of octopus this way.

1 medium-large octopus (800g–1kg cleaned weight)

50ml olive oil

1 onion, finely chopped

1 teaspoon harissa
(a Tunisian hot pepper paste – use more if you enjoy very spicy food)

1 tablespoon tomato purée

1 tablespoon cumin seeds, roasted in a hot pan and then pounded

1. Braise or boil the octopus, making sure you reserve either the liquid that emerges during braising, or the water in which the octopus has been boiled.

2. Cut the octopus into smallish pieces.

3. Heat the olive oil in a pan large enough to take all the ingredients and add the onion to colour.

4. Add the octopus pieces, the harissa and the tomato purée and sauté briefly before adding a cup of the reserved octopus juices.

5. When the liquid has all but evaporated add enough of the octopus juices to cover the contents, cover the pan and simmer slowly for about an hour.

6. Add the roasted and ground cumin seeds and simmer for 15 minutes before serving.

The roasting and grinding of the cumin seeds makes a huge difference. Use ready ground cumin if you must, but it will have nothing like the same flavour.

Tunisian Dried Octopus and Pasta Stew

Although you have to plan a day ahead to soak the legumes and octopus, the recipe is then fairly quick to prepare.

100g dried chickpeas

100g dried broad beans (fava beans)

200g dried octopus

75ml olive oil

1 large onion, sliced

1 stick celery, chopped

4 medium carrots, peeled and chopped

3 turnips, peeled and chopped

2 cloves garlic, finely chopped

25g flat-leaf parsley, chopped

2 tablespoons tomato purée

1 tablespoon harissa paste

2 teaspoons paprika powder

1 teaspoon cumin seeds (briefly toasted in a dry pan)

salt

500g orzo or quadrettini pasta

2 lemons

1. Soak the chickpeas and broad beans in water overnight. Do the same with the octopus (in a separate bowl).

2. Heat the oil in a large heavy-bottomed pan over medium heat. Sauté the onion until golden, stirring regularly, about 20 minutes. Cut the octopus into bite-sized pieces and add to the pan, along with the chickpeas, broad beans, celery, carrots, turnips, garlic and 20g of the parsley and sauté for another minute.

3. Next, add the tomato purée, harissa, paprika, cumin and some salt, and continue sautéing for a few minutes. Add 1.5 litres of water, and simmer until the vegetables are tender.

4. Add the pasta, and continue simmering until al dente.

5. Adjust the seasoning, and add lemon juice to taste. Serve, garnished with the remaining parsley, and lemon wedges on the side. Couscous would be the perfect accompaniment.

Takoyaki

This recipe is only included for the benefit of those who possess a *takoyaki* griddle.

Make a batter mix (150g flour, 1 litre water, 4 eggs). Heat a *takoyaki* griddle and brush lightly with oil. Fill each indentation with batter and then drop in a 1 cm cube of pre-cooked octopus, some red pickled ginger (*beni shoga*), a few rice crispies, a 1 cm cube of blanched *konnyaku* (taro) and some chopped spring onion. Once the bottom is cooked, carefully turn the dumplings. Keep turning until crisp on the outside but still soft at the centre. Serve brushed with a little soy sauce and garnished with finely shaved bonito flakes (*hana katsuobushi*) and dried seaweed powder (*aonori*).

BABY OCTOPUS RECIPES

Baby octopus (which can be adults of small species or juveniles of larger species) are usually very tender, and can be cooked very briefly. If they do become rubbery, it is almost always because they have been cooked for too long. Baby octopus can be stir-fried, thrown directly on the barbecue for a quick char, or flash-grilled – all without pre-cooking.

Deep-fried Baby Octopus

This is a variation on the classic salt-and-pepper squid. Deep-frying works well for baby octopus, cooking them quickly, evenly, and keeping them moist. The coriander flavour is best if you grind it yourself: briefly toast some coriander seeds in a dry pan over medium-high heat until fragrant, then grind in a spice grinder or pestle-and-mortar. The use of corn-flour rather than ordinary flour gives a more crunchy texture. These go well with a dipping sauce – try sweet Thai chilli sauce, or homemade tartare sauce.

500g cleaned baby octopus

30ml Thai fish sauce

30ml lemon juice

2 teaspoons ground coriander

2 teaspoons paprika

1 teaspoons cayenne powder

15g fine sea salt

2 teaspoons freshly-ground white pepper

350g corn-flour, sifted

oil for deep frying

coriander leaves, for garnish

lemon, cut into wedges

1. Mix the fish sauce and lemon juice in a bowl. Cut the baby octopus into bite-sized pieces and add to the bowl. Marinate in a cool place for about an hour.

2. Mix all of the dry ingredients together in a bowl.

3. Remove the octopus from the marinade and drain well. Add the octopus pieces to the spice mixture. Transfer to a sieve or colander and shake well to remove excess flour.

4. Heat oil in a deep-fryer or deep pan to 190°C and fry the octopus for 1–2 minutes until the coating is crisp and the octopus tender.

5. Drain on paper towels. Garnish with chopped coriander, and serve with lemon wedges.

For a more European take on this deep-fried recipe, simply omit the marinade at stage 1 and coat with seasoned flour before frying. These deep-fried baby octopus are delicious as part of an Italian-inspired *fritto misto*, with other deep-fried delicacies such as squid, prawns, scallops, small fish.

Grilled Thai Baby Octopus with Mango

The ginger and fresh chilli zing in this dish combines perfectly with the caramelised octopus and sweetness of the mango. It also makes a perfect barbecue dish.

250g cleaned baby octopus

50ml dark soy sauce (the thicker and sweeter variety, called *laochou* in China)

1 mango (not too ripe; best is one of the Thai green eating varieties)

20g coriander leaves, whole with stems removed

1 long red chilli, seeds and pith removed and thinly sliced

4 spring onions, white and light green parts only, thinly sliced

10g mint leaves (about 20 leaves), cut into chiffonade, reserving a few whole leaves for garnish

For the dressing:

juice from 2 limes

1 tablespoons Thai fish sauce (*nam pla*)

2 teaspoons finely grated ginger

1 teaspoons chilli powder or cayenne

2 tablespoons Thai sweet chilli sauce

2 hot green chillies, seeds and pith removed and finely chopped

1. Combine all the dressing ingredients and mix well. Adjust seasoning, then set aside.

2. Blanch the octopus then drain well on paper towels.

3. Brush the octopus with the soy sauce. Cook under a hot grill, turning once or twice, until the octopus has caramelised to a light golden-brown.

4. Cut the mango flesh into small cubes. Add the coriander leaves, red chilli, spring onion, octopus, and chiffonade mint leaves. Add the dressing and mix well. Garnish with a few whole mint leaves and serve.

Korean Spicy Octopus Stir-Fry (Nak-ji Bokum)

Koreans love spicy food, and this dish can really bring tears to the eyes. Feel free to tone down the spice a little.

800g cleaned baby octopus (about 12)
20ml vegetable oil
1 medium onion, thinly sliced
60g carrot, thinly sliced
3 fresh (hot) chillies, thinly sliced
3 spring onions, white and light green parts only, sliced
salt
a few mint leaves and coriander leaves for garnish
For the marinade:
6 shiitake mushrooms, quartered
20g garlic, finely chopped
50g *kochujang* (Korean chilli paste)
20g hot chilli flakes
20ml soy sauce
20g honey
20ml sesame oil
15g toasted sesame seeds
120ml water

1. Mix together all the marinade ingredients. Cut the baby octopus into bite-sized pieces, and add to the marinade. Leave in a cool place for about an hour.

2. Heat 20ml vegetable oil in a pan over medium heat. Sauté the onion for a few minutes until it is translucent, add carrot and fresh chillies and continue sautéing for a few more minutes until the vegetables have softened. Add the spring onion and sauté for another minute.

3. Add the octopus with its marinade, stir and cover. Simmer until the octopus is just cooked (5–10 minutes, depending on the thickness of the pieces; they should be able to be easily pierced with a fork).

4. Adjust the seasoning, and garnish with chopped mint and coriander leaves. Serve with steamed Japanese rice.

Pickled Octopus

Pickled octopus is a popular dish all over the Mediterranean, and a great way to preserve extra cooked octopus – perfect for using up the mantles, say, when a recipe calls only for the arms.

cooked octopus (about 500g)

1 tablespoon coriander seeds

½ teaspoon black peppercorns

red wine vinegar (about 500ml)

2 hot red chillies

4 cloves garlic (whole, peeled)

a 5 cm piece of lemon peel

4 bay leaves

1 teaspoon dried oregano

½ teaspoon sea salt

extra-virgin olive oil

1. Cut the cooked octopus into bite-sized pieces and put into a pickling jar that will hold them comfortably.

2. Place a dry pan over medium heat and toast the coriander seeds and peppercorns, stirring or shaking the pan regularly, until they are fragrant. Take the pan off the heat, continuing to shake while it cools a little. Add 200ml vinegar (be careful: if the pan is too hot, the vinegar will give off strong fumes), chillies, garlic, lemon peel, bay leaves, oregano and salt.

3. Place the pan over a high heat, and bring to a simmer, stirring occasionally. Once the vinegar is simmering, remove from the heat. Add an additional 200ml vinegar, cover and allow to cool to room temperature. (Heating only half of the vinegar makes this quicker; if you want to further speed up the process, you can cool the vinegar mixture in an ice bath.)

4. Pour the cooled vinegar mixture and aromatics over the octopus, ensuring that the octopus pieces are just covered. Top up with additional vinegar if necessary. Add a layer of olive oil at least 1cm deep, then refrigerate. Allow to marinate for at least a week before using. The octopus can be kept for up to 3 months.

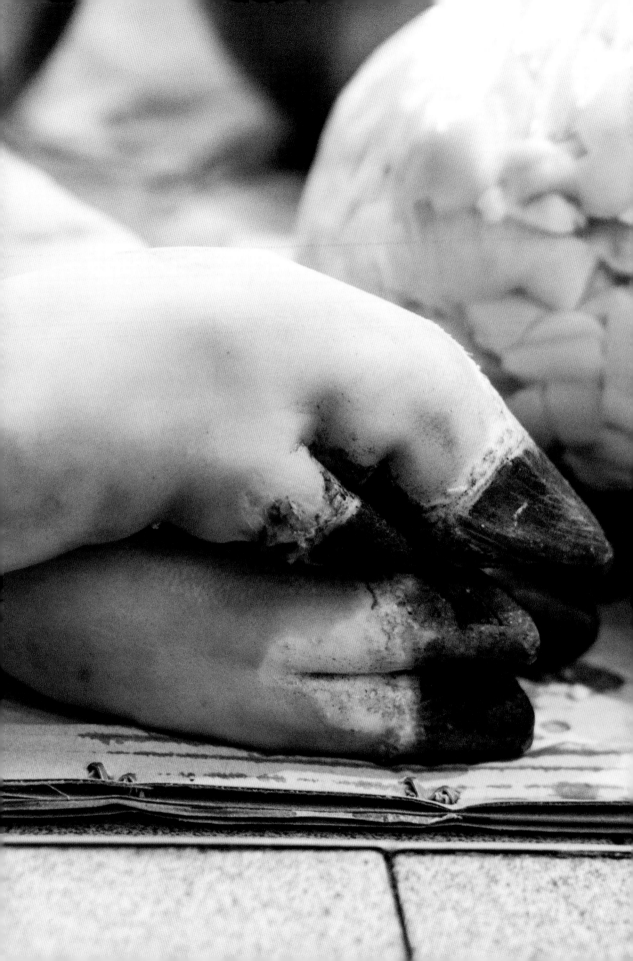

3. CHEEKS AND FEET

The food of kings

The *berline*, little more than a heavy sedan chair supported on four wheels and drawn by two pairs of horses, rocks and rolls along the barely made road. The King is not used to discomfort, but he is acutely aware that there is no time to lose. If everything goes to plan, tomorrow he and his entourage will be at the Royalist stronghold of Montmédy, where he will raise an army with the help of his brother-in-law the King of Austria. His plan – well, truth be told, his wife's plan – is a desperate one. The French royal court abhors the way Louis' perceived indecision compounds their own, ever-worsening, situation. But his loyal subjects love him, and he prays they will understand that he simply has to crush the revolution. Hours earlier, at the royal residence in Les Tuileries, he left a proclamation for the Jacobin revolutionary leaders. The constitutional monarchy the National Assembly have coerced him into, he wrote, is leading France toward 'absolute anarchy'.

The year is 1789. It is the early hours of 21 June, and the road in question runs between Châlon-en-Champagne and Verdun in the Argonne region of north-eastern France. Louis is tired and hungry. Soon the *berline* will arrive in Ste. Ménéhould, where it will leave the main road and turn north onto a track leading through the Argonne Forest all the way to the castle at Montmédy.

The King muses:

> My Grandfather was le Roi-Soleil; his rights were divinely bestowed and mine are too; yet here I am dressed as a valet. The King and the Queen will not go hungry.

He calls his instructions down to the driver.

The driver pulls the coach in at a small restaurant in the sleepy town, and a short plump man wearing an ill-fitting valet's costume steps down leaving the family governess, disguised as a wealthy baroness, to look after the children. Marie-Antoinette, dressed as a humble maid (or, as some reports claim, a baker), steps down too. Together they walk into the restaurant. The castle, full of Leopold's men and loyal emigrées, is only hours away, but Louis XVI has only one thing on his mind: crisp, fine, honey-coloured breadcrumbs encasing a single tender, gelatinous pig's trotter which has been cooked so gently, and for so long, that even the bones have yielded to a chewy softness – Pied de Cochon Ste. Ménéhould.

But Pied de Cochon is also a food of the people. A fierce republican war veteran serving as the local postmaster in Ste. Ménéhould – Jean-Baptiste Drouet – is also in the restaurant. He greets the valet and maid as they enter and watches them take their seats next to a huge stone fireplace where no fire has burned for weeks. He continues to eat but the more he watches them, the more his interest is piqued. There is something unconvincing about them: the inappropriate way they address the proprietor; the way the scruffy valet sits bolt upright; the way the maid – for she is only a humble maid – dabs at her mouth with a serviette after each and every mouthful. Both of them possess a bearing that belies their status.

The valet turns for a second and Drouet sees him for a moment in profile. Something clicks. In his pouch he has a single golden *ecu*, which he places into the palm of his hand under the table. He compares the profile of the man on one side of the coin with the man on the other side of the room and rises slowly, leaving through the back door.

Barely half an hour after the coach has left Ste. Ménéhould, Louis is woken from his postprandial nap as the coach is stopped at the bridge over the Meuse at Varennes.

It will not be the last time a man lost his head over a dish of trotters. Vive la République!

Drouet was offered a considerable reward for his quick thinking, which – so legend has it – he refused. He later became a key figure in the 'Convention', Danton and Robespierre's revolutionary legislative assembly, which operated through the Committee of Public Safety. Ever the moderate, Drouet also proposed the slaughter of all British residents in France during the French Revolutionary Wars.

The restaurant at Le Cheval Rouge, 1 Rue Chanzy, Ste. Ménéhould, 51800, still serves the famous dish on their €29 *formule*, and it's only €10 in the brasserie there. (They also have rooms and pretty hanging baskets.) Not far away, the Hotel de la Poste has an engraved picture of the king's *berline* on its front window. Drouet was a postmaster, but we have no idea whether this is the place the king stopped (the recipe is actually attributed to a chef at the now defunct Hotel de Metz, and, anyway, neither of us have eaten there). But they also serve Pied de Cochon, as do many other restaurants, brasseries and *charcuteries* in the town, and if you visit in May, you can attend the Fête du Pied de Cochon.

It's a neat story, though we wouldn't testify in front of a grand jury that it isn't apocryphal. But one thing is certain: if you were to ask a hundred individuals to come up with their Top Ten 'Food of Kings', we would put money on the humble pigs trotter not appearing once. Our money would go on the usual suspects: caviar, truffles, foie gras, and such like.

No one would have raised an eyebrow had Marie Antoinette uttered 'Let them eat trotters.'

Despite the lowly status of the trotter, it – and other humble ingredients such as ox and pigs cheeks, cow-heel, snout – have over the years acquired a good deal of kudos, and become *trés chic* in many top restaurants. French culinary legend Pierre Koffman famously marries the humble trotter with a stuffing of chicken mousseline, sweetbreads and morels. Thomas Keller's own recipe for trotter and hock terrine slices pan-fried in panko crumbs and served with *sauce grebiche* would have been right up Louis XVI's street.

But we hope you agree it is odd that while those who can afford it enjoy such humble ingredients in the rarefied atmosphere of starred restaurants, where a huge white plate is presented to the diner under a giant silver cloche, to be lifted from the plate in grand ceremonial style (at precisely the same time as your dining partner, of course), the ingredients themselves are rarely seen in our supermarkets. We perfectly understand that they don't regularly stock beluga caviar or fresh white truffles, but trotters? And what's even stranger is that, considering how cheap, delicious and easy to prepare they are, many people would not consider buying them even if they were.

Why are people in the UK only prepared to eat trotters if they are paying through the nose for it? We suspect – partly at least – that it is something to do with a version of the mystique that surrounds unfamiliar ingredients in general. We mentioned this in our chapter on the octopus: it is a bizarre, mystical beast, which therefore demands to be cooked using bizarre, mystical methods. Trotters fall into a similar camp: compared to the ubiquitous chop or tenderloin, they are perceived as looking strange and unappealing. Only a culinary high priest is equipped with the requisite training, technique and talent to turn such a thing into something edible.

The thing is that's not true. Yes, most of the ingredients we discuss in this chapter take a long time to cook but it's not as if you have to be standing over the stove watching each strand of collagen break down. You'll spend much more time at the stovetop tending a risotto for 20 minutes (plus 5 to allow the rice to *manticare*) than you will if you stew ox cheeks in red wine for 5 hours. Indeed, legend has it that the Ste. Ménéhould recipe was created by accident, when a chef forgot about the trotters he was simmering in stock and left them overnight! With feet and cheeks, as we shall see, the secret is long and slow.

In 1986, a small group of demonstrators including journalist and political activist Carlo Petrini gathered to protest peacefully against the proposed opening of new McDonalds restaurant in the centre of Rome. A few years later, you may recall, French farmer Josć Bové and 300 colleagues would dismantle a partially constructed McDonalds in Millau, France. (As a result of Bové's imprisonment, angry farmers dumped 6 tonnes of manure at a McDonalds in Arles.) But that was not Petrini's style: the demonstration in Rome was an entirely good-natured one. He decided to fight the onslaught of fast food by setting up a non-profit food and wine organisation called Arcigola. Then, in the late 1980s, he and a group of like-minded colleagues signed the 'Slow Food Manifesto'. A movement was born, it's aim to 'prevent the disappearance of local food cultures and traditions, counteract the rise of fast life and combat people's dwindling interest in the food they eat.' The movement is now established in 160 countries with over a million members, and millions of people support their activities, which include campaigns to raise awareness of food sustainability issues, protect local produce and retain, and increase, biodiversity and encourage people to (re)discover overlooked, undercooked ingredients. We share their aims, and applaud both their ethos and their energies. You should certainly join the Slow Food network, wherever you live.

Cook ugly! Cook slow!

Face facts

Female members of the French nobility in the late 1700s would have shared roughly the same skin-care routine: apply rouge and make-up liberally in the morning; reapply during the evening; leave on overnight; wake up and reapply a fresh layer in the morning, ensuring that any spots, pimples or open sores are well covered. Personal hygiene was not high on anyone's agenda at the time. Most people (even members of the nobility) bathed once a month at most, and toilet habits also left a lot to be desired. There were commodes here and there, but many visitors to the Palace at Versailles relieved themselves at, shall we say, their own convenience. Anywhere. The scale, grandeur and sheer beauty of the Palace and Gardens are overwhelming even to the modern visitor. But the fact remains that in the 1700s Versailles stank

Versailles was a vast cesspool, reeking of filth and befouled with ordure. The odour clung to clothes, wigs, even undergarments. Worst of all, beggars, servants, and aristocratic visitors alike used the stairs, the corridors, any out-of-the-way place to relieve themselves.

M-L Gothien, *History of Garden Art,* 1913

Which makes Marie Antoinette's approach to her *toilette* all the more revolutionary. Marie cleansed her face every morning, in an *eau cosmetique* made from a range of fruit and herbs, camphor, bread, white wine and, among other ingredients, stewed pigeons. After that, she would apply an astringent toner and whitener. Marie also bathed frequently, exfoliating her skin with bran and cleansing herself with soaps scented with amber and bergamot. As well as this, and probably as a means of keeping the Versailles stench at bay, she insisted on constantly dousing herself with orange blossom water, and wherever she went there were containers of *pot pourri*, pouches of perfume and fresh flowers.

Had it not been for the fact that they signalled for her the beginning of the end, Marie would have been delighted had she known that those final mouthfuls of Pied de Cochon Ste. Ménéhould probably benefited her complexion at least as much as her pigeon water cleanser. In 2009 a team of Japanese scientists from Tokyo University (M. Tanaka, Y. Koyama and Y. Nomura) suggested that eating collagen peptides – trotters are high in collagen – reduces the effects of sun-related skin aging. An article in *Gourmet* magazine in the US entitled 'Collagen Cuisine' described how the trend has caught on in Japan over the past five years or so and there is now a huge market there for collagen capsules, collagen drinks and even pink grapefruit flavoured collagen marshmallows. Japanese ramen eateries proudly announce that their noodles contain twice the normal amount of collagen. In February 2011, a highly fashionable restaurant in north London announced a menu featuring a series of collagen-rich dishes entitled 'Eat yourself Beautiful'. Forget botox injections, keep your skin wrinkle-free by lunching on a 'collagen inside out dumpling', followed by 'clear soup of chicken, wild rice and collagen jelly', then 'collagen and seaweed salad'. Wash the whole thing down with a collagen cocktail.

Ingestible collagen has been big business in China for centuries and the unlikely source of the best raw material is donkey skin, which is soaked and stewed to produce *ejiao*, or donkey-hide gelatin. *Ejiao* is available for sale in biltong-like sticks, which can be chewed, or in sachets, which are steeped in boiling water to make a collagen rich drink. Beijing restaurant Wang Pang Zi Donkey Burger serves up a range of collagen rich dishes, including donkey penis burgers, sautéed donkey hide, spiced donkey pastries and donkey soup.

It is sometimes claimed that Japanese (and other Asian women) age better than their European counterparts. We are agnostic on this issue, but if it is true, it might just be down to that daily dose of ass-hide glue (as *ejiao* is sometimes translated). The science is being done, and time will tell.

Neither of us speaks Cantonese, but we assert with complete confidence that *ejiao* is pronounced 'eeyore'.

Chic science

This book aims to inspire you to celebrate forgotten or underrated foodstuffs, and this chapter aims to show you how to prepare cheeks and feet expertly. We explain below why they are so amenable to slow-cooking: because of where they originate in the animal's body they are high in connective tissue that is full of collagen – this collagen can only be gelatinised, and hence tenderised, by long exposure to low heat. Once you've tasted pigs cheeks, for example, we doubt you'll ever go back to the ubiquitous 'chop', which can be so dry and flavourless. The Boeuf Bourguignon you cook with ox cheeks will be the best you've ever tasted. And you don't have to stuff pigs trotters with veal sweetbreads and morels to create a delicious supper (though if you have some sweetbreads and morels, we suggest you do). Trotters are delicious stuffed with mashed potato, or, added to a stew of any kind, provide a wonderfully unctuous sauce. Award-winning British chef and writer Fergus Henderson makes a gelatinous concoction called 'trotter gear' from trotters, vegetables and Madeira. A jar or two of trotter gear is a permanent fixture in our refrigerators, and lends depth and texture to casseroles, pies, soups and stews.

Understanding how cooking affects various cuts of meat is important to getting tasty, tender results, so here's a brief explanation. Muscles are made up of bundles of proteins ('fibres') laid out in parallel, which give the meat a noticeable grain. Tough connective tissue holds these bundles together and connects them to bones. Muscles also contain fat, which stores energy.

Different muscles in different parts of the animal are designed to perform different functions, and have different combinations of muscle fibre, connective tissue and fat. Leg muscles, for example, need to carry heavy loads, so have lots of connective tissue. This makes them tough. Similarly, cheek muscles do the heavy, repetitive work of chewing, so are also tough – think of a cow chewing the cud all day long. Muscles that do less work, like the back and the loin, have less connective tissue and are consequently less tough.

Fat can be located alongside muscle, as fatty tissue (fat cells in a matrix of collagen); or, it can be spread throughout the muscle, which is known as 'marbling'. Marbling is an indication that a muscle is doing a lot of work, and needs a ready supply of energy. Thus, marbling is a sign of toughness – and the fat cells themselves are held together by collagen. However, melted fat lubricates the meat as we chew it, which gives the feeling of more succulent and slightly more tender meat. This, together with the fact that fat also carries a lot of flavour, is why highly marbled meat is so prized.

Connective tissue within muscles is made up mostly of collagen, which is too tough for us to easily bite through. If heated for long enough and at high enough temperatures, however, the protein bundles in collagen break down into single strands – or denature – to form soft, unctuous gelatine. The tough sinews that connect muscle to bone are made up of different proteins (reticulin and elastin), which can only be denatured after very long cooking and/or near-boiling temperatures.

When meat is cooked, the proteins change in important ways. When heated to about 40°C to 50°C, the muscle proteins begin to denature. The meat becomes more dense, and tougher. Above 50°C, collagen begins to shrink, squeezing out more meat juices, and also starts denaturing to form gelatine, increasing the tenderness. The higher the temperature, the greater the shrinkage and the faster the collagen becomes gelatine.

This explains why some cuts of meat are suited to long, slow cooking whereas others are best cooked quickly. Tough meat with lots of connective tissue becomes tender after a long time, as the collagen turns gradually into gelatine. These cuts benefit from braising – cooking in a liquid – so that they don't become too dry as a result of moisture loss from collagen shrinkage. On the other hand, tender cuts of meat become dry and tough if cooked for a long time, because they lose their juices, but there is not enough collagen to produce succulent gelatine. They are best cooked quickly, to minimise collagen shrinkage and hence moisture loss.

All cuts of meat benefit from browning – briefly searing the outside at very high temperature. This does not 'seal in the juices' as sometimes claimed. Rather, it produces rich flavours and aromas via the Malliard reaction – a complex and not completely understood chemical reaction that creates the characteristic roast meat flavour (if it was understood better, food scientists would be able to create convincing roast beef flavour crisps). In normal circumstances, the Malliard reaction only really gets going above 120°C, a temperature that is hard to reach on the surface of a moist cut of meat without overcooking the inside. This is why chefs brown meat in small batches, in very hot pans and with plenty of oil; or sear steaks on extremely hot grills; or resort to using deep-fryers or blow-torches. But don't over-do it: if the temperature gets too high, you'll end up with bitter charcoal rather than pleasant roast. (Pressure cookers also produce high enough temperatures for the Malliard reaction to take place, and as long as they don't boil dry, there's no risk of burning.)

RECIPES

All recipes serve 4 unless otherwise noted.

Daube de Boeuf Bourguignon

In our chapter on octopus we provide a recipe for J. B. Reboul's octopus 'en daube'. The Provençal *daube* is also often made with beef, and what follows is the version made slightly further north, in Burgundy. In truth, it can be prepared using any cheap cut of beef – ox-tail is also good – but we have found that by far the best results are obtained using ox cheeks. Happily, this option is also the cheapest. If you're planning on serving this dish on, say, Saturday, then marinate the meat overnight from Thursday evening and cook on Friday. Up to a point, the flavour improves each time the dish is warmed up, so you could begin the marinating process up to 4 or 5 days ahead.

2kg ox cheeks

1 onion, roughly chopped

1 carrot, roughly chopped

1 stick celery, roughly chopped

1 head of garlic (split in two around the equator, rather than the poles)

fresh thyme

bay leaf

1 bottle of good red wine
(burgundy is traditional, but any good red is suitable – though remember that if it isn't good enough to drink, it isn't good enough to cook with)

olive oil

500ml water (better still, chicken or veal stock)

salt and freshly-ground black pepper

1. Cut each ox cheek into two pieces.

2. Place all the vegetables and herbs in a large bowl and pour over the red wine; leave overnight in a cool place.

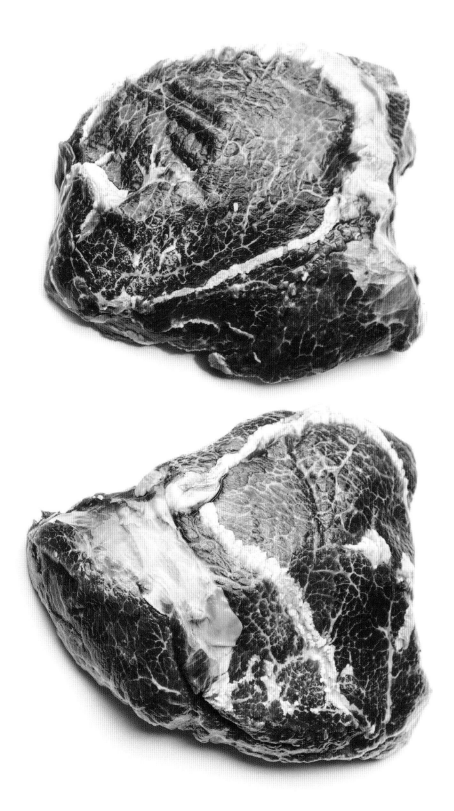

3. Pass the marinade through a sieve. Reserve the solids and reduce the wine by half over a high heat.

4. Brown the meat in hot olive oil in batches (use plenty of oil and do not crowd the pan). Remove the meat from the pan, then brown the vegetables also. Return everything to the pan, including the wine reduction, and add 500ml of water or stock. Season with salt and pepper, and bring back to the boil.

5. Cover with a cartouche made with greaseproof paper, and a lid.

6. Cook in a slow oven (150°C) for 3–4 hours.

We like to cook this in the evening and after the required cooking time simply turn off the oven and leave the *daube* to cook even more slowly overnight in the cooling oven. In the morning, remove the *daube* (it will probably still be slightly warm), transfer it into another container and refrigerate. About half an hour before it's time to eat, reheat the dish gently, adjust seasoning and serve with mashed potato. The meat will have reached the point of tenderness the French call *à la cuillère* (literal meaning 'with a spoon') – it should just fall apart.

Cooking (with) Wine

With very few exceptions, wine needs to be cooked in order that some (or most) of the alcohol is boiled away. It can also be flamed off, by igniting the alcohol as the wine comes to a simmer. This is more than just visual showmanship (or pyromania) – the flaming process reduces acidic flavours.

Some people say that slow cooking meat in wine helps denature the protein bundles in the collagen (effectively tenderising it), but for us whether or not you use wine in your cooking depends on whether you like the taste of it. We do (very much), and for that reason we never cook with wine if it isn't good enough to drink. Avoid so-called cooking wine at all costs.

Daube options:

• When you take the dish out of the oven, remove the cooked vegetables and blitz them with a little of the meat juice in a blender – this makes the sauce even thicker.

• Before serving add lardons of bacon, button mushrooms and baby onions or…

• … a tablespoon of sauce made with finely chopped garlic, parsley, anchovies, capers, lemon and extra virgin olive oil.

- Any leftover *daube* makes a wonderful sauce to dress pasta a few days later.

Once you have this recipe in your repertoire, you effectively have dozens. Here are a few adaptations:

- You can use pigs cheeks instead of ox and many recipes tend to substitute white wine for the red wine, or even cider. In Donostia (San Sebastian, Spain), they cook their pigs cheeks in red wine. We've tried it, and, having tried it, we doubt we'll go back to white again (so substitute pigs cheeks for the ox cheeks and proceed exactly as above).

- If you do stick with white wine, then to your pigs cheeks add belly pork, black pudding and chorizo, potatoes, cabbage and chick peas – hey presto, *cocido Madrileño*!

- You can also cook the *daube* with veal cheeks (if you don't like the idea of veal, see box on page 71), but if you do, we recommend using half red wine and half Madeira in the marinade. Serve with a nice creamy polenta.

- Lamb shanks or shoulder are cooked beautifully this way, although the cooking time can be reduced considerably.

- The vegetables can, of course, be adapted to suit the season; in our experience, *daube* is more suited to cold days when you need something warming, but at the end of summer, as the nights are shortening, some ripe tomatoes would be lovely, fennel also.

- The alcohol in the dish can also be changed. Stout or port (or a mixture of the two) changes the dish in interesting ways. Elizabeth David gives an eighteenth-century recipe from one William Verral, then chef of The White Hart Hotel in Lewes, in which beef is cooked in stout and port. Verral was promoting what he called the 'French method' of cooking and the dish is delicious. The White Hart Hotel is still there opposite Lewes Crown Court, with the same largely Elizabethan interior. Alas, despite the fact that it still claims to serve 'classic French fare', on our last visit there was very little method on display, French or otherwise.

Ox-Cheek Salad à la Hongroise

That most modern cars are fitted with Global Positioning Systems (for pre-GPS, biblical navigation techniques, see the *Book of Ezekiel* 21:21 – quoted on page 224) has deprived twenty-first-century motorists of one of the most exciting, enjoyable and – dare we say – fundamental aspects of any kind of travel: that is, the possibility of arriving in a place you hadn't been intending to travel to. One of us recalls a potentially calamitous misread of the map in the mid-80s, which sent our Citroën 2CV heading due east on French 'N' roads instead of due south (the direction we thought we were going). Yet it led to an unforgettable evening meal, in a hotel in the middle of we-still-don't-know-where, comprised of the most amazing lake perch fillets fried in butter and unforgettable chilled red Bugey.

The proprietor also distilled his own *digestif*, which, alas, ensured we lost even more time the following morning. Analogously, the preferred modern day method of ordering books/e-books online, and, in particular, only doing so when you have found precisely what you are looking for, deprives people in no small way of the pleasure to be found in wandering around a library or a bookshop not knowing what it is you are looking for at all. Chance is not to be underestimated. Had it not been for one of us wandering into an old bookshop many years ago, and happening upon Alfred Suzanne's *A Book of Salads: The Art of Salad Dressing* – translated by A. Garance and 'revised and augmented' by C. Herman Senn MBE – we would never have been able to share with you this delicious recipe for ox-cheek salad.

1kg cooked ox cheeks
(pressure cook them in beef stock for 45 minutes or, alternatively, cook as for a *daube*, above)
250g waxy potatoes, cut into 1 cm dice
250g celeriac, cut into 1 cm dice
250g beetroot, cut into 1 cm dice
a handful of capers
vinaigrette made with red wine vinegar and olive oil in a 1:4 ratio, mustard to taste, seasoned well with salt and freshly-ground black pepper

1. Shred the meat with your fingers while it is still warm.

2. Blanch the potatoes, celeriac and beetroot separately in boiling salted water for 5 minutes.

3. Combine the warm meat and vegetables in a bowl. Toss gently with vinaigrette and capers.

The operative word is 'gently' here. If you agitate the mixture too much, the colour from the beetroot (which will bleed a little of its juice out anyway) will overly dominate the visual appearance of the dish. Jerusalem artichoke would make a nice substitute for either the potato or the celeriac.

Veal Ethics

The mere mention of the word 'veal' is usually enough to raise the hackles of even the most committed omnivores. As an ingredient veal is almost universally rejected in the UK. There are two reasons. Firstly, those doleful, long-lashed eyes, those little wet noses and spindly Bambi legs mean calves are just too cute to eat: we hope we have dealt with that argument in our opening chapter. Secondly, veal production, people argue, is an utterly inhumane practice.

Let's elaborate briefly on the second point. In the 1980s, the practice of rearing veal calves in crates so tiny they couldn't even turn around, in total darkness, and then transporting them live in those crates, on journeys that lasted as long as 40 hours, attracted widespread – and justified – public condemnation. The purpose of the crates, which are still used in the US and parts of Europe, is to render the calves immobile; immobility ensures minimal muscle development, and muscles that are undeveloped make for the tenderest meat. Recall from above that those muscles that work hardest for an animal result in the toughest meat.

To say that opposition to live veal exports became something of a *cause célèbre* is an understatement. Sussex police were at one point forced to employ an extra 1,000 officers on a daily basis to repel protesters. The 'Battle of Brightlingsea' – a sustained ten-month campaign by protesters and local residents to prevent the export of live calves from the small Essex port (which was being used because the major ferry operators were by now refusing to transport live animals) – was the scene of fierce fighting between protesters and the police, who had resorted to using riot control methods. As a result of news being leaked of the sale of calves from his farm, the Minister for Agriculture William Waldegrave received death threats; letter bombs were delivered to several export companies.

Veal crates were banned in the UK in 1991, but the export of veal calves continued. In 1993 alone, the UK exported half a million calves to satisfy the massive demand for veal in continental Europe. With the advent of 'mad cow disease' in the late nineties, however, the market collapsed.

Thank goodness for that, we hear you say. Now all those pretty calves can live happily ever after.

Er, no. One of us comes from a family of dairy farmers, so allow us to provide a brief overview.

In order that a dairy cow can keep producing milk, it needs to calve fairly regularly: around every year to fourteen months. If the calf that is born is female, then all is well: she can go on to become a dairy cow just like her mother. But if the calf is male, it's a whole other story. The male offspring of dairy cows are, in effect, a by-product of the dairy industry, so if you are a vegetarian, but you drink milk, or eat cream or cheese, then this concerns you too. The male calves make virtually nothing at markets in the UK and the meat from adult dairy bulls is sub-standard: these animals are not, after all, raised to be meat, they're raised to produce milk, and the price a farmer would receive for an adult dairy bull would not even recoup their costs in feed and care.

So what happens? Well, what happens, more often than not, is that male calves are simply shot, an hour or so after birth. The situation is cruel, and wasteful in the extreme.

As a result, many frustrated, but enterprising dairy farmers have begun to seek ethical ways in which to raise calves for consumption as veal. 'Rose-veal', as it is known in the UK, is now available in many major UK supermarkets and has the backing of the RSPCA's 'Freedom Food' campaign and 'Compassion in World Farming'. Eat veal.

THREE RECIPES FOR HEADS

Head Salad

Had we decided to write a different kind of cookbook, we might have christened this dish *tête de veau* (*agneau*, *cochon*) vinaigrette or *testina di vitello* (*agnello*, *maiale*) *insalata*, and included a heavily saturated colour plate of the dish, garnished with cubes of jelly and, for luck, a glistening slice of black truffle.

But this is *Ugly Food*, so 'head salad' it is – calf, lamb or pig.

1 head

1 onion, chopped

1 stick of celery, chopped

1 carrot, chopped

1 bay leaf

Vinaigrette:

100ml extra virgin olive oil

30ml red wine vinegar

Dijon mustard (some brands sell a mustard/horseradish blend which we find to be excellent for this recipe)

chopped parsley, dill and celery leaves (enough to give you a handful)

salt and freshly-ground black pepper

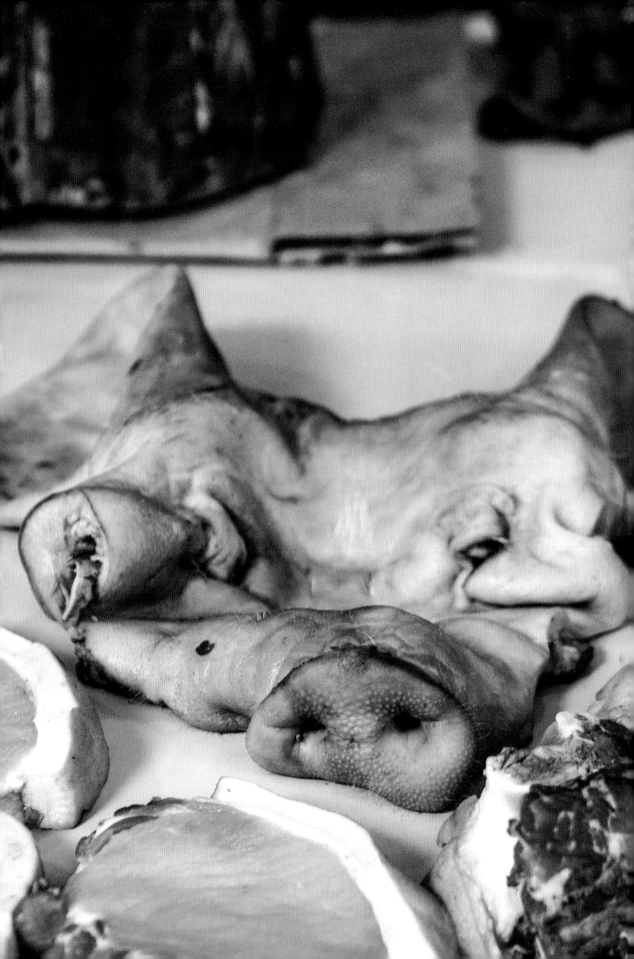

1. Place the head in a large pan, cover with water and bring to the boil; simmer for 10 minutes and then discard the water.

2. Rinse out the pan, fill with fresh water and add all the other ingredients; add the head and simmer for an hour and a half (or until you can see the meat falling off the bone); remove the head from the liquid (and save the liquid – it will enrich your next stew beyond belief).

3. Remove all the meat from the head and rip it into small shreds with your fingers; refrigerate.

4. Place all the vinaigrette ingredients in an old jam jar; replace the lid and shake well for a minute until you have a smooth, creamy sauce.

5. Dress the meat with the vinaigrette and serve with fresh bread.

In his wonderful book *Nose to Tail Eating*, Fergus Henderson includes a delicious recipe for Warm Pig's Head Salad. Proceed as above, removing the meat from the skull and shred with your fingers whilst warm. Do not, however, refrigerate. Instead, toss immediately with plenty of wild rocket or watercress, sorrel leaves (if you can get them – better still grow them), curly parsley, cubes of yesterday's bread, chopped cornichons and capers. Dress with vinaigrette made from olive oil, red wine vinegar, mustard, chopped garlic, salt and pepper.

In typical style, Henderson adds a subtle extra touch that elevates the salad to another level. That is, remove the ears before boiling the head and when they are done (which will be before the rest of the head) remove them and let them cool. Just before serving the salad, slice the ears very thinly and cook them in a deep fryer, being careful to keep them moving in the oil so they don't clump together. Drain the ears on kitchen paper and top your warm salad with the crisp ears. Perfect.

Calf's Head Madrilène

A typically beguiling recipe from Edouard de Pomiane, who introduces it as follows:

> I ate this dish in Madrid and it charmed me, so I shall tell you about it.

Pomiane's recipe calls for a boiled, boned calf's head, but you can just as easily begin with a whole head as in the previous recipe. Don't, however, refrigerate the meat once you've taken it off the bone. It wants to be served warm.

cooked calf's head meat, torn into shreds

80g tomato purée

2 cloves of garlic, chopped

generous slug of extra virgin olive oil

40g salted capers, soaked in water for 15 minutes

black olives

4 hard-boiled eggs

parsley

1. In a small saucepan, heat the tomato purée with enough water to thin it to a syrupy consistency.

2. Add the garlic, olive oil, capers and olives and cook gently for 10 minutes or so.

3. Add the calf's head meat and keep it warm.

4. Place the meat and sauce on a serving platter and surround with quarters of hard-boiled egg; sprinkle with parsley and serve.

Whilst it's not in de Pomiane's recipe, we sometimes add fillets of anchovy to the sauce (or strew them over the eggs). We find it adds an interesting further savoury dimension.

Boiled Sheep's Head

This is a traditional Scandinavian dish, known as *smalahove* in Norway and *svið* in Iceland. Unlike the previous recipes, the split head is served as is on the plate, which can be a little challenging for the uninitiated. This book is really not about extreme food; we include the recipe because we believe it is important to eat the whole beast, and because it really is very tasty – cheeks, tongue and other morsels all on a single plate. In the same vein, this dish is normally served without the brain, but your head will probably come with it, and it would be a shame to waste it, so we provide a tasty recipe for that too.

The traditional method is as follows. Take one sheep's head (serves 2). Burn away the wool, leaving the skin intact and browned. Split the head in two lengthways with an axe or bone saw and remove the brain. Clean the split head under running water, paying particular attention to the ears and eyes. Salt it, and leave to dry for several days, then smoke over alder or juniper. The split head is then placed in a pot and covered with water, brought to the boil, skimmed, then simmered, covered, for 60–90 minutes until the meat is cooked through but still holding to the bone. It is served hot with mashed swede and boiled potatoes, accompanied by aquavit.

In the UK and the rest of the European Union, heads from sheep over one year old are banned due to concerns about the prion disease scrapie (although there is no evidence that scrapie has ever been transmitted to humans). Here is a recipe using lambs heads instead. Your pot will need to be fairly large in diameter. Also, invite your guests to eat the ears and their surrounds and the flesh around the eye sockets first, as this is the fattiest and best when hot. Then move on to the cheeks, tongue and all the rest. The eyeballs are traditionally reserved for last.

2 lambs' heads, cleaned and split
(preferably singed not skinned so the ears remain on)

For the rhubarb chutney:

400g red onion, medium dice
60g butter
300g rhubarb, cut into 2cm lengths
1 star anise, whole
60ml red wine vinegar
20g caster sugar
salt

1. Carefully remove the brains (if included) and reserve for the recipe below.

2. Place the split heads in a pan of generously salted water large enough to fit them comfortably. Bring to the boil and skim. Cover and simmer for 60–90 minutes until the meat is cooked through but not yet falling off the bone.

3. Meanwhile, make the rhubarb chutney. Sauté the red onion in the butter for a minute or two, then add the rhubarb and star anise. Simmer gently for 15 minutes, stirring occasionally. Add the vinegar, sugar and salt and simmer a further 15 minutes until soft and gooey.

4. When the heads are ready, remove and allow to drain briefly. Serve with the rhubarb chutney and Hamburg parsley mash (recipe, p. 213). Some aquavit would also be good.

Here's one way to prepare the brain, again inspired by Fergus Henderson, which would be a nice starter while the heads are cooking. We think you should try – it really does have an appealing taste, and the texture is fabulous.

Sheep's Brain on Toast

reserved lamb's brain lobes

1 onion, medium dice

1 carrot, medium dice

1 leek, white and light green parts, medium dice

4 cloves of garlic, crushed

bouquet garni
(8 peppercorns, bay leaf and thyme sprig, tied in muslin or leek leaves)

slices of toasted bread

extra virgin olive oil

fleur de sel or Maldon salt

sprig of flat-leaf parsley, leaves chopped

1. Add the vegetables and bouquet garni to a pan of lightly salted water and simmer for 15 minutes.

2. Rinse the brain lobes in cold water and remove any membrane or veins. Carefully lower into the pot, and simmer gently for 8 minutes. Remove with a slotted spoon and leave to cool.

3. When the lobes are cold, slice lengthwise and arrange on slices of toasted bread garnished with olive oil, salt and parsley.

Bath Chaps

The boning out and rolling of heads (as mentioned in an earlier recipe) appears to be a dying art. Bath chaps are a speciality of the West Country, they used to be quite common, but are now much harder to find. Downland Free Range Meat in Melksham, Wiltshire still sell them, though; you can find them online. Basically, the boned out head is rolled around the tongue, then brined and (sometimes) smoked. Once you get it home, you boil it for 2 hours or so and then let it go cold. Serve with a simple green salad dressed with the vinaigrette for head salad above.

Char Siu Pigs Cheeks

This is delicious with rice, or noodles, and makes a great filling for soft bread rolls.

1kg pigs cheeks

For the marinade:

50ml dark soy sauce

50ml hoisin sauce

50ml mirin

25ml sesame oil

25g sugar

25ml honey

2 cloves of garlic, finely chopped

30g fresh ginger root, grated

1. Mix the marinade ingredients together. Place in a ziplock bag and add the cheeks; marinate overnight in the fridge.

2. When the time comes to cook, pre-heat your oven to about 160°C; you'll need a tray with a rack, the grill pan for example.

3. Fill the tray with boiling water and place the cheeks on the rack above the water. Keep the marinade.

4. Pop into the oven and cook for as long as it takes for the pork to become a deep, appetising colour and meltingly tender (3–4 hours is normal); keep checking the level of water in the tray, but try and ensure that when the pork is cooked, the liquid has reduced considerably (if it reduces too quickly, add a little more water).

5. At this stage add the remaining marinade into the tray and cook it on the hob until it is syrupy; add the pork to the thick sauce and leave to cool.

Chopping Parsley

When chopping parsley, use absolutely the sharpest knife you have to avoid bruising rather than chopping; you'll know if you've bruised the parsley rather than chopped it because your chopping board will be bright green when you've finished. Unless you plan on eating your chopping board, it probably doesn't make sense to leave all the flavour behind on it.

Anglerfish (or Cod) Cheeks with Bacon

As we remarked earlier, the head of the anglerfish hardly ever makes it to the fishmonger's slab. It's a shame for two reasons: firstly, they make a delicious soup; secondly, the cheeks are the tenderest, most delicate flesh on the whole fish. Cod cheeks are also delicious. If you do happen to get hold of either type of cheek, simply wrap them in a thin slice of bacon, hold it in place with a toothpick and fry gently in a mixture of oil and butter.

Hake Cheeks with Salsa Verde

500g hake cheeks, skin on
450ml extra virgin olive oil
4 cloves garlic, finely chopped
large bunch of parsley, finely chopped
juice of 1 lemon
salt

1. Place the hake cheeks (in Basque, they are called *kokotsxas*) skin side up in the olive oil in a large pan.

2. Raise the heat slowly to a temperature which is almost too hot for you to put your finger in, but not quite.

3. Slowly cook the cheeks – you will notice that the olive oil thickens slightly (which is because the cheeks are releasing their gelatine).

4. After 10 minutes, put the garlic, most of the parsley and the lemon juice into a small pan; add a couple of ladlefuls of the warm cooking oil to the pan and season well with salt.

5. Serve the cheeks on a white platter, dress with the flavoured oil mixture and add a further sprinkling of parsley.

If you are lucky enough to take a trip to Donastia you may well come across this dish as one of the pintxos – or tapas – you are served in one of the many bars. If you are seriously lucky, you will manage to get a table at a certain establishment in Calle de Guetaria, which is in the basement of one such tapas bar. The restaurant takes reservations, but only reluctantly, and is open weekday lunchtimes only. The short, perfect menu includes Kokotsxas with salsa verde and a selection of other Basque dishes.

Tonbridge Brawn

Without doubt one of the finest cookery books ever written is *Modern Cookery for Private Families* by Eliza Acton, first published in 1845. Not to put too fine a point on it, but it is infinitely better than Mrs Beeton's much more well-known *Book of Household Management*. The latter was published two years after Acton's death in 1859 and plagiarises Acton's earlier work shamelessly.

We don't know whether the town of Tonbridge in Kent is still famous for brawn (Frank Dean's Butchers of Goring, West Sussex, certainly is, and will sell you a slice or two of the most delicious brawn if you're ever passing) but below we present a step-by-step, albeit not entirely faithful, version of Acton's delicious recipe. Acton's version includes saltpetre, the use of which is now restricted, so we make the recipe without and it is very successful. The other difference between our recipe and Acton's is that she instructs you to split the pig's head first, and remove the brain and all bones before cooking. We find that boiling the head first, and then removing brain and bones is easier.

1 pigs head
2 pigs trotters
red wine vinegar
2 heads of garlic
2 onions
2 sticks of celery
4 cloves
2 bay leaves
sea salt

1. Put the head and trotters into a deep, capacious pan and cover with water and a generous splash of red wine vinegar.

2. Add all the vegetables plus the cloves and bay leaves and bring the pan to a very gentle simmer.

3. After an hour, you will find that you can pull off the ears; do so and set them to one side.

4. After 2–3 hours, you'll notice that the cheeks are beginning to fall off the bone. At this stage, remove the head and trotters from the cooking liquid. Strain the cooking liquid, discarding the vegetables and aromatics, and return the liquid to the heat. Reduce it by about half and salt very well.

5. Don't be tempted to wait until the head and trotters have cooled completely; while they are still warm, pick through all the meat from the head – the cheeks, the snout, the tongue, the lot – and remove the meat from the trotters.

6. Line a terrine mould with cling film and fill with the meat; cover with your reduced liquid until the terrine is full; make sure there are no pockets of air lurking under the meat.

7. Leave it overnight in the fridge and remove an hour or so before serving (depending on the weather); it doesn't want to be fridge cold, but neither should it be warm.

Acton recommends serving this with an Oxford Brawn Sauce. We quote her recipe:

> Mingle thoroughly a tablespoonful of brown sugar with a tea-spoonful of made mustard, a third as much of salt, some pepper, from three to four tablespoonsful of very fine salad-oil, and two of strong vinegar; or apportion the same ingredients otherwise to the taste.

We like this sauce a lot. We also like it with Opie's pickled walnuts (in fact, the pickling juice of these walnuts tastes a little like Acton's sauce – though it has no oil in it).

The Greeks make brawn – they call it *pictí* – by boiling the pigs head in water with bay leaves and black peppercorns. Instead of vinegar, large quantities of lemon juice are added to the stock before it is poured over the meat to set.

Whole Roast Fish Heads

This is a fantastic dish – tasty, thrifty and simple – and the charred heads with herbs look simply beautiful. Keep the heads from smaller fish for stock (along with the bones and off-cuts) and use larger heads for this dish. As with buying any fish, make sure the heads are fresh, with bright eyes and deep red gills.

Two heads from decent-sized (3-4 kg) white fish should be enough for four people; we recommend coley or pollack over the less-sustainable cod and ling (though if you have found sustainable cod and ling, they would be perfect too).

2 decent-sized fish heads including gills and collars (the part between the gills and pectoral fins)

4 cloves of garlic, cut into thin batons

thyme sprigs

6 bay leaves

salt and freshly-ground black pepper

1. Rinse and dry the heads, then rub with olive oil.

2. Using a larding needle or point of a paring knife, cut a dozen or so small slits in the fleshy parts of each head and insert half the garlic and half the thyme (reserving the other half). Tuck a bay leaf into each gill and mouth.

3. Place in a baking tray, and scatter over the remaining garlic and thyme, along with plenty of salt and freshly-ground black pepper.

4. Roast at 220°C until cooked through (about 30 minutes, depending on the size of the heads).

5. Serve, accompanied with boiled potatoes and the juices from the pan poured over the heads.

Crappit Heids

Many fish will arrive at your local fishmonger's (and certainly at your local supermarket) already cleaned and gutted. But if you do get the chance to buy half a dozen locally caught cod or haddock, we'd urge you to try this recipe from the Isle of Lewis. It's to be found in F. Marion McNeill's wonderful book *The Scots Kitchen*. We approached this recipe with a deal of scepticism, but to say we were pleasantly surprised with the results would be an understatement. Ms McNeill really knew what she was doing. The list of ingredients is short, but the end product is simply amazing. Of this recipe, McNeill quotes Alistair Hislop's (1875) *Book of Scottish Anecdote*: he describes it as 'a sort of piscatorial haggis'.

heads and livers of haddock or cod

oatmeal

salt and freshly-ground black pepper

a little milk

1. Chop the livers finely.

2. Mix with an equal weight of oatmeal.

3. Season (very) well and bind with milk.

4. Stuff the heads with the mixture.

5. Place the heads at the bottom of a buttered pan in which they fit tightly, cover with water and poach gently for half an hour.

6. Serve with mashed potato (or neeps and tatties).

McNeill observes that 'modern' crappit heads (she was writing in the 1930s) had replaced the traditional stuffing with one of crab or lobster, mixed with ship's biscuit, anchovy and egg yolk. We haven't tried this, more luxurious, version, but our gut feeling is that putting lobster in crappit heids offends the MAXIM OF PURITY about as much as adding langouste to *bouillabaisse*.

The stock produced by cooking the liver-stuffed heads is superb: it is rich, flavoursome and wonderfully unctuous. You shouldn't throw away the liquid in which you cook fish. Learn to love its texture and flavour. If you've prepared it from fresh fish, it will freeze perfectly well and form the basis for countless other dishes. Alternatively, pop it in a jar and put it in your fridge next to your trotter gear.

In honour of Fergus Henderson, we name this particular essence 'Heid Gear' (to be worn at your peril).

Alexis Soyer's Toad-in-the-Hole

Alexis Soyer was one of the first celebrity chefs. Having left France in 1830, he came to England to work as a chef for numerous private families and, in 1837, became Head Chef at the Reform Club. His 'Lamb Cutlets Reform', a dish of savoury breadcrumb-encased lamb chops, is still on the menu there. During his lifetime, Soyer devoted much of his time to charitable causes, including setting up a soup kitchen to help victims of the Irish famine, and the publication of a number of books intended to improve modest home cookery. Among the latter was his famous volume *A Shilling Cookery for the People*. We're not entirely sure whether nowadays you could get away with a book containing a chapter entitled 'General Ignorance of the Poor in Cooking', but we'll be generous: his heart seems to have been in the right place.

Nowadays, toad-in-the-hole usually involves sausages baked in the oven in a thick batter, but Soyer gives this brief version using ox-cheek and sheep's heads:

> Ox cheek and sheep's heads, previously cooked and nicely seasoned, with the addition of a little chopped onions added to the batter, is an economical dish. A few slices of cooked potato may be added.

Soyer's batter recipe is as follows:

1. Put 6 tablespoons of flour into a bowl.

2. Add 4 eggs, salt and pepper.

3. Add one pint of milk and mix until very smooth.

You may have your own recipe for batter. We prefer one made with half milk and half beer, which is a little lighter, and some people fold whisked egg-whites into the batter to make it super-light. In general, we prefer our hole less soufflé-like.

Out of nothing more than curiosity, we also provide a version of Soyer's toad-in-the-hole made with sparrows. We have never tried this, but in the interest of providing tasty, sustainable alternatives to brine-injected chicken breasts, here goes:

1. Take twelve, freshly plucked sparrows. (Soyer says nothing about whether or not they should have been cleaned, but we presume so).

2. Wrap each sparrow in a rasher of bacon and hold this in place with a toothpick (alternatively, thread several birds on to metal skewers); pack the birds relatively tightly into a shallow baking dish.

3. Cover with batter and bake in a low to moderate oven for 2 hours.

The tradition of netting and eating small birds – sparrows, thrushes, larks, warblers, and even blackbirds – lives on in large parts of continental Europe. Since he was probably brought up with this tradition, Soyer would have regarded this recipe as a perfectly thrifty way of using a fairly commonly available ingredient. We doubt, however, that many people in the UK would actually have taken the time to cook it. It seems to us to be another example of a deeply culturally entrenched Anglo Saxon view that there is something inherently barbaric about the whole process. One journalist writing in a 2000 article in the *Irish Times* put it like this:

> Not that anyone wants to adopt the French attitude to what may be killed and eaten and what not. The French are the French. Leave it at that.

Ah, yes. The French. Name one food-related thing they have ever done for us? We wonder if the journalist in question has ever consumed a battery-bred chicken? If so, he has engaged in behaviour infinitely more barbaric than the netting and eating of wild birds. If the birds in question are protected or endangered, of course, that's a very different thing.

Incidentally, Soyer suggests that in the absence of sparrows (imagine) half a dozen larks might be substituted. Since the population of larks in the UK has fallen by 75 per cent in the past 40 years, we implore you not to heed his advice. Blackbird-in-the-hole, anyone?

Corned Beef

Thanks in the main to the ubiquity of canned corned beef this ingredient is much maligned in the UK. But it's just salted beef (the 'corned' part of the name refers to the fact that large kernels of sea-salt used to be referred to as 'corns') and is fabulous cold with pickles or hot with mashed potato. This recipe below calls for ox cheeks, but any cheap cut of beef would work well.

2kg ox cheeks
100g sea salt
50g caster sugar
1.5 litres water
2 pigs trotters

1. Mix together the salt, sugar and the water; heat it and stir until all the solids have dissolved and then set aside to cool. (If you want to do so quickly, dissolve the salt and sugar in half the amount of water, and cool the brine by adding 750g of ice cubes.)

2. Once cool add the beef and leave to soak for three days.

3. On the fourth day, remove the beef, discard the brine and rinse the meat well under running water.

4. Place the meat in a large pan with the trotters and cover with cold water; bring to the boil and simmer for 3 hours, or until the cheek meat gives way when you touch it with a wooden spoon.

5. Remove the meat from the water and set the trotters aside to use in another recipe (see below).

6. Bring the liquid to the boil and reduce it over a high heat until reduced by about half (you need approximately 600ml).

7. Either chop the meat as finely as you can with a knife or, if you have a mincer, mince through a large plate (between 5 and 10 mm).

8. Mix the chopped meat with the reduced cooking liquor (most of which should be absorbed, leaving you with a relatively loose texture); taste for salt and add a generous number of turns of black pepper.

9. Place the mixture in a terrine and leave to set in the fridge overnight; you can weight it down if you want, but we prefer a looser consistency.

Pigs Trotters Braised in Sweet Vinegar

This Cantonese dish is the ultimate comfort food. In China, post-partum mothers traditionally eat it during their so-called 'confinement' period, the weeks in which they stay at home after the arrival of a new baby. It's incredibly cheap and nutritious, and tasty too.

2 pigs trotters prepared as above and cut into bite-sized pieces – in general, there's more meat on the front trotters, but the back trotters give you more collagen and unctuousness

500g of fresh root ginger

a generous slug of sesame oil

400ml sweet Chinese black vinegar

400ml black rice vinegar (sometimes known as *zhe jiang* vinegar)

150g light muscovado sugar

(the final amount you need will depend on the exact nature of the mix of vinegars that you use – a sweeter mix will require less sugar)

1. Slice the ginger and fry gently in the sesame oil.

2. Add the trotters and get them well-acquainted with the ginger and sesame oil.

Preparing feet for cooking

If your trotters require chopping, we find it is easier to get the butcher to do this. Chopped feet are a more fiddly to prepare, it's true, but trotters are not easy to chop and domestic kitchens sometimes lack the cleavers (and brute force) required. It's your call.

Before actually cooking your trotters (or, for that matter, ears or tails), you should carry out the following procedures:

1. Clean the feet well. With pig and sheep trotters (or calves' feet) this might involve the use of a blowtorch, or naked flame of some kind, to singe any remaining hair before removing. In the absence of a blowtorch we have had success with a disposable razor, but have also found that being discovered in the bathroom lovingly shaving a pig's trotter can be hard to explain.

In the case of poultry feet, blanch the feet for 1 minute and remove the outer skin. (Exactly as you would if you were skinning tomatoes.)

2. Parboil the trotters or feet for 5 minutes in well-salted water. This removes any remaining traces of dirt or blood.

Proceed with recipe.

3. Add the vinegar, sugar and water to cover.

4. Bring to the boil, cover the pan and cook very slowly for no less than 3 and up to 5 hours (it works best to put the dish in a low oven).

5. Serve piping hot.

We like to make this dish a couple of days before we eat it; this gives the flavours time to mature. Traditionally, peeled hard-boiled eggs are added to the final dish. When the trotter and ginger have all been eaten, don't throw away the vinegar. If you boil it up every few days and skim, it will keep for about a month and makes a wonderful condiment to add to wintry stews or drizzle over rice.

Sheep's Trotters with Avgolemono

Avgolemono is a delicious sauce made from egg yolks – the Greek word for eggs is αυγό (avgo) – and lemons. We first ate this dish in Greece, although the first time we had it, we simply couldn't believe it was trotters. Greeks waste nothing, and – as far as we could tell – pretty much every meat dish served in the small taverna in which we ate was lamb-based (including the head that was served up on the table next to us).

lamb or sheep's trotters (about 12)

juice of one lemon

3 egg yolks, whisked

salt and freshly-ground black pepper

a court bouillon made with two chopped celery stalks, one chopped onion, one fincly chopped carrot, black peppercorns and water

1. Having cleaned and parboiled your trotters as below, cook them slowly in the court bouillon until the meat is literally falling off the bones.

2. Remove all the meat from the bones and shred into thin pieces.

3. Add about 500ml of the strained cooking liquid to a saucepan and add the meat.

4. Before serving, place the pan over a low heat to warm through if necessary. Pour off 100ml of the warm cooking liquid from the pan into a mixing bowl and add the lemon juice and egg yolks, mixing vigorously so that the egg yolks thicken the liquid and turn it a delicate yellow colour (you don't want the yolks to form cooked strands, you want them to amalgamate into a sauce). Pour it back into the pan.

5. Season well and serve with crusty bread.

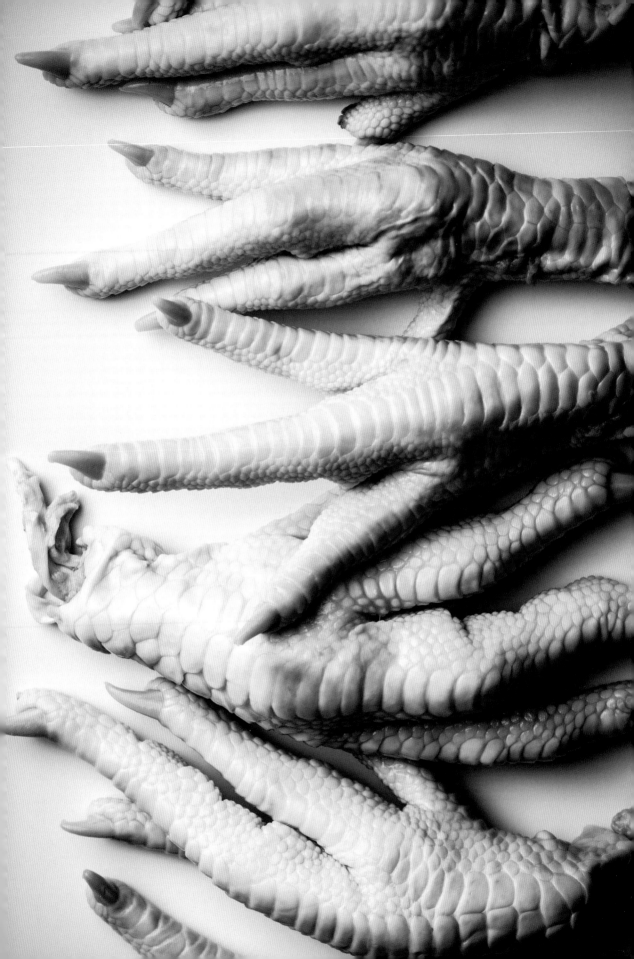

Chicken Feet Braised in Hoisin Sauce

The word 'hoisin' has its origins in the Cantonese word for seafood. However, it contains no seafood ingredients at all (moreover, its sweet, salty taste makes it an ideal complement to meat rather than fish). This dish is wonderful as a light lunch served with rice, or as one dish forming part of a larger meal.

1kg prepared chicken feet (see box on page 86)

30g knob of fresh ginger root

1 clove garlic

40ml hoisin sauce

20ml soy sauce

40ml Chinese rice wine or dry sherry

20g sugar

60ml oil

20ml cornflour, mixed into enough water to make a thick paste

1. Boil the chicken feet in water for 1.5–2 hours, so they're almost tender.

2. Grate the ginger and garlic, then combine all the ingredients apart from the chicken feet and cornflour mixture in a bowl.

3. Heat the oil In frying pan or wok and add the feet, stirring well.

4. Add the hoisin mixture to the pan and let it bubble and thicken for 5 minutes (the feet will go nicely brown).

5. Add some water, cover and reduce the heat; simmer for 30-45 minutes.

6. Before serving, thicken the sauce with the cornflour and water mixture.

Deep-fried chicken feet are delicious too. Make sure they are well cooked (so 2 hours minimum). Simply dip in egg, then flour, then egg, then flour again and deep fry at 180°C. Serve with Thai sweet chilli sauce or any oriental dipping sauce.

Lao Chicken Feet Salad

500g prepared chicken feet (see box on page 86)

100g red shallots, thinly sliced

100g cucumber, cut in half lengthways and sliced on an angle

30g galangal (or ginger) cut into thin batons

half a stalk of lemongrass, white part only, thinly sliced
1 spring onion, thinly sliced
handful of mint and coriander leaves, mixed

For the dressing:

2 Thai chillies (bird's eye chilli), roughly chopped
1 clove garlic, roughly chopped
20g caster sugar
40ml lime juice
20ml fish sauce
20ml fermented fish sauce (*nam pla raa*)

1. Blanch the chicken feet by simmering in lightly salted water for about 15 minutes. Drain and allow to cool completely.

2. De-bone the feet. First, snip off the tips of each toe. Then, with the foot facing upwards, slice down the centre of each toe all the way to the middle of the foot, and down the centre of the foot to the leg end. Carefully remove the leg bone and all the toe bones and joints, trying to leave the skin as intact as possible. We won't lie: this is fiddly. You can, however, do it in advance.

3. Make the dressing. First, pound the chopped chillies and garlic in a mortar a little to break them up, then incorporate the sugar. There should still be some chunks of chilli. Gradually add half of the liquid ingredients. Taste for seasoning: it should be hot, salty, sour and a little sweet, with no single taste dominating. Add more fish sauce, fermented fish sauce and lime juice to achieve a good balance.

4. Shred the de-boned feet lengthwise into half-centimetre strips. Combine with the vegetables and herbs. Toss with the dressing.

5. Serve, together with white rice – or even better, sticky rice.

Insalata di Nervetti

This delicious salad is a speciality of Lombardy. The combination of the rich, mild and slightly fatty calf foot with the fresh, crunchy onion and pepper reminds us of the Salata do Polvo on page 40. Begin the dish the day before you intend to eat it.

2.5kg of prepared calves' feet (see box on page 86)

court bouillon made with water, an onion stuck with cloves, a chopped
carrot and two sticks of chopped celery
50g red onion
50g red pepper
a generous splash of extra virgin olive oil
a rather less generous splash of white wine vinegar
parsley
salt and freshly-ground black pepper

1. Poach the calves' feet gently in the court bouillon for anything up to 3 hours; the meat should be coming away from the bones.

2. Tear the meat into fine shreds and place it in a large bowl or terrine dish; barely cover with the bouillon, check the seasoning and allow to cool.

3. Cover the terrine with a lid and put it in a cool place for a few hours. You will notice when it begins to set; once this starts to happen, weight it down with something – try to keep it in a cool place but out of the fridge.

4. In the morning your *nervetti* will resemble brawn somewhat; slice it finely and place in a bowl.

5. Slice the onion and pepper as finely as possible and add them to the *nervetti*; add the olive oil and white wine vinegar and mix well.

6. Sprinkle with chopped parsley and serve.

We haven't specified the quantities of oil and vinegar, but while you should be more restrained with the vinegar than the oil, you should aim to use slightly more vinegar than you would in a normal vinaigrette. The feet are slightly fatty and the vinegar offsets that nicely. This is also a good way of using preserved red peppers, or even red peppers you have roasted and skinned. However, if you do this, use a slightly larger proportion of red onions: preserved or roasted peppers don't add the same texture as fresh ones. For a slightly more meaty, less gelatinous *nervetti*, use one calf trotter and a veal shank, or a quantity of stewing veal.

Silk Purse Salad

Our book is all about challenging certain cultural assumptions, so here goes.

500g prepared pigs ears
2 star anise
30g root ginger, finely sliced

2 large carrots, 3 spring onions and 1 cucumber cut into fine strips
(all well chilled in the fridge)

125ml Chinese plum sauce

1 red chilli

splash of soy sauce

sugar

lemon juice

toasted sesame seeds

a small bunch of coriander

1. Prepare the ears according to the instructions on preparing feet (see box on page 86).

2. Return the well-rinsed ears to a pan of cold water with the star anise and the finely sliced ginger; cook for 45 minutes until the ears are tender.

3. Remove the ears and chill.

4. Slice the ears very thinly and mix them with the chilled strips of carrots (kohlrabi works fine too), spring onions and cucumber; toss the meat and vegetables in the plum sauce and add some finely sliced pieces of red chilli.

5. Season with soy sauce, lemon juice (and a little sugar if necessary).

6. Top with toasted sesame seeds and chopped coriander.

You can, you know. As this salad proves.

Pieds de Cochons Ste. Ménéhould

Full disclosure. We have never eaten a version of this dish in which we found the bones so soft that they could comfortably be eaten, but that could be lack of breeding (see introduction to this chapter). Notwithstanding that, this is a delicious, and incredibly cheap starter or light lunch dish. We have found (and tried) a range of recipes, but the following, adapted from *French Provincial Cooking* is our favourite. The key may lie in the initial salting.

4 pigs trotters

1 onion

1 carrot

a bunch of parsley

a stick of celery

a bay leaf

a slice of lemon

For the final coating:

200g dry breadcrumbs

200g melted butter

1. The day (or even 2 days) before cooking, prepare the trotters (see box on page 86), then sprinkle coarse sea salt over them and leave them in a cool place.

2. On the day of cooking, place them in a pan with the vegetables and lemon, cover with water and bring to a simmer. Remove any scum that forms (though there won't be much, due to the earlier blanching), cover the pan so that no air can escape (a tea towel between pan and lid is a good technique). Simmer gently for 4–5 hours, or until, when you take a peek, the meat is coming away from the bones.

3. Remove the trotters from the liquid, which you should treasure. Either freeze it or put it in jars. It will add the most sensational flavour and body to any stew or gravy you make.

4. Allow the trotters to cool a little but while they are still warm, roll them in melted butter and then breadcrumbs. They want to be well coated. Elizabeth David recommends 40g each of butter and breadcrumbs per trotter, but we have, on occasion, used more. The quantity in the recipe reflects this.

5. Place the trotters in an oven pre-heated to 220°C and leave them in there until the exterior is a chestnut brown and crisp. Serve them on hot plates and provide a large helping of remoulade sauce (recipe on page 210) and a little bitter green salad to accompany.

If, for whatever reason, the thought of eating this dish occurs to you whilst you are fleeing across Europe from enemies who would not think twice about removing your head, we recommend you reach safety first and then send for a take-out.

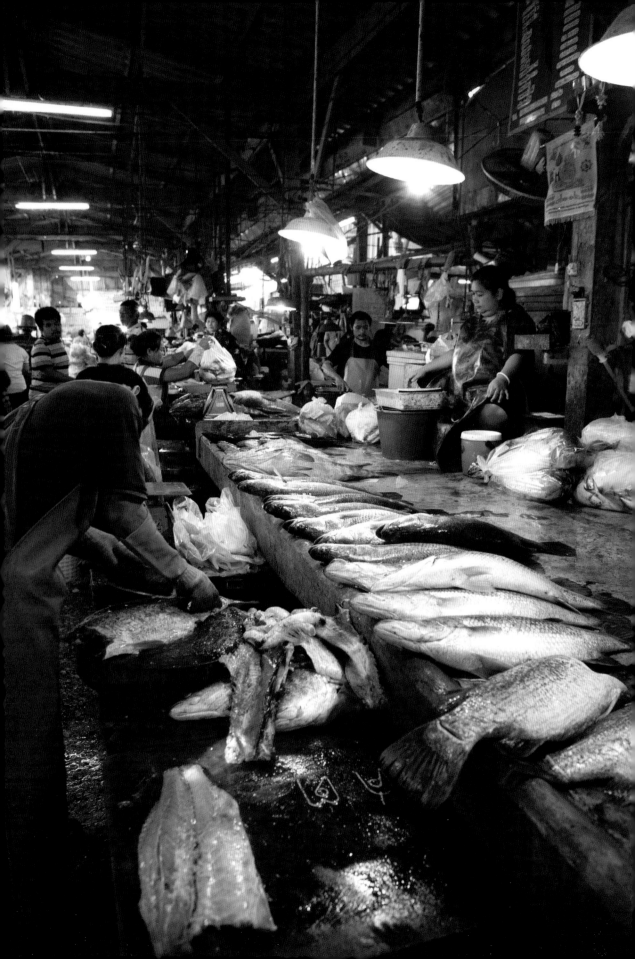

4. UGLY FISH

Sea robin

> Among the fish that may be classed as edible, but which are entirely neglected...
> is the sea robin, grunter or gurnard. This curious, but rather forbidding creature, is,
> in reality, one of the most delicate morsels that can be laid before an epicure, the
> flesh being snow-white, firm, and really as good as that of king-fish, or whiting. In
> fact, it would be hard to distinguish them when placed on the table.
>
> J. Carson Brevoor, quoted in G. Goode, *The Fisheries and Fishery Industries
> of the United States*, 1884

Twelve-year-old girls, it seems, are particularly susceptible to the culturally
entrenched fears of food that perpetuate in the Anglo-Saxon world. The girl
in question is a fussy eater, just the kind of person whose horizons our book
aims to expand. She loves her crumbed fish, but it has to be the plain old
'white' stuff from the piles of neat fillets on the slab.

We decided to perform an experiment.

A local fisherman, who still lands his boats on the beach in the town in
which one of us lives, had come back from a night's fishing with a few codling,
some mackerel, a couple of sea bass, one or two cuttlefish and a huge catch of
gurnard ('sea robin' in the US, sometimes 'gurnet' in the UK). Now the gurnard
is not a pretty fish. It is about one-third head, and that head possesses a huge
mouth and jutting lower jaw that gives the fish an unflattering, rather gormless
expression. The lower rays of the pectoral fins, the 'wings' just behind either
side of the head, extend downwards separately below the head to help the
fish forage for food, giving the impression of whiskers clinging to its chin (the
gurnard is sometimes known as the 'pig-fish', a reference to the grunting sound
they make once caught – the word 'gurnard' is probably onomatopoeic). The
bodies are often greyish brown in colour, but many in UK waters have a tinge

of red about them. If the sea bass is an elegant, streamlined silver sports car, glinting in the sunlight, the gurnard is a rusting truck scavenging for scraps along the seabed.

Anyway, we bought half a dozen for next-to-nothing, to gasps of derision and disgusted facial contortions from the person behind us in the queue, filleted them – easily done – and froze the heads, racks and some of the flesh to make a delicious fish soup or stew in the weeks to come. The rest of the flesh we skinned, floured, egged, crumbed and served to the subject of the experiment. She absolutely loved it, and once we had told her about the fish she had eaten, and about the environmental implications of continuing to eat vulnerable species such as Atlantic cod, she declared gurnard 'the best fish in the world'.

How many of you can say she's wrong?

Not many, we would guess. Because British fish consumers typically regard ugly fish such as the gurnard with the same degree of suspicion, even disdain, as they do the octopus. They're just too ugly to eat. Many fishermen in the UK regard gurnard as nothing more than lobster-pot bait. Indeed, with fish the problem goes deeper: many shoppers who turn their nose up at ugly fish actually seem to believe that fish which is edible should not even look like fish at all, hence the rise in popularity of the faceless fillet, or the cuboid fish-'brick' in the freezer cabinet.

In the UK, that monster of the deep the anglerfish, usually sold as 'monkfish', is considered so ugly that its head never even makes it on to the fishmonger's slab. Strictly speaking, 'monkfish' is the term for the meat of the angel sharks – *squatina squatina* and *squatina dumerili* – which, since they became critically endangered in 2010, are now no longer marketed. (And even when they were, angel shark was more likely to be found in the form of crumbed 'scampi' in the freezer cabinet than fresh on the fishmonger's slab as monkfish.) As we have pointed out a number of times, there seems to be something peculiarly Anglo-Saxon about this kind of extreme reaction to ingredients perceived in any way as unusual or unfamiliar. The Spanish and Portuguese happily present anglerfish – known as *rape* or *tamboril* – in its glorious entirety, knowing that the beasts with the fattest cheeks will be fought over by discriminating customers (and if you've never tasted anglerfish liver, you haven't lived). In France the *grondin* (gurnard) is prized.

In the fish markets of South-East Asia, consumers would not be remotely interested in seeing fillets of soft white flesh which, to be honest, could have their origins in any one of a hundred different types of fish. They want to see the fish itself, because the whole fish is a much better guide when it comes to accurately gauging freshness and quality. You're buying fish, so why would you not want it to look like fish?

In this chapter we'd like to try and encourage you to change the way you think about fish generally: to see ugly fish in a different way (perhaps even as 'cute', a view taken by one of our daughters – though as we have discussed earlier, there's much more behind our food preferences than cuteness and ugliness). Our ultimate aim is to convince you to go out and buy them, and buy them whole, or at least – if you have them filleted – to keep the heads and bones. Once you have finished this chapter, we hope that not only will you know a great deal more about fish and fish cookery in general, but will also experiment freely and regularly with these wonderfully tasty and economical ingredients, despite the fact that they are, well, ugly.

Why? Well, while this chapter is about ugly fish, it is – we think – a chapter with noble aims. We have good reason for recommending that you modify your fish-shopping and fish-eating habits. The sea is being over-exploited. In certain areas, stocks of fish are critically endangered. If we don't stop, or at the very least, seriously reduce fishing for species such as Atlantic cod, tuna, haddock, salmon, eel, orange roughey, (so-called) 'hoki' (actually the deep-sea rat-tail) and red snapper, these fish will become commercially extinct, possibly extinct full-stop.

The solution to this problem, you might think, is simple: fishermen need to adopt more selective fishing methods, to stop landing those species that aren't sustainable and start landing those that are. The sea is swimming with species of fish that are delicious to eat and perfectly sustainable, so why don't the fishermen target them? There is a straightforward answer. You won't eat them!

You can't blame the fishermen. They target the species they know will sell at market, and the wholesalers at the market buy and sell snapper, Atlantic cod, tuna and so on because they know that they are the fish that we, the consumers, want.

Many of the ugly fish that are the subject of this chapter are cheap, sustainable and absolutely delicious. In North Atlantic waters, for example, there are – among others – gurnard, John Dory, huss (dogfish), conger eel, garfish (with their alarming blue-green bones), eel-pout and members of the cod family not generally considered as good for eating – the tomcod, the so-called poor cod and pollack. Our recipes include two favourites eaten a great deal on the Atlantic coast of Portugal, the stone-bass, wreck-fish or cherne, and the scad or horse mackerel. No Mediterranean fish soup is complete without rascasse, a goggle-eyed, spiny red thing that looks like an armour-plated gurnard on steroids (more sea Rambo than sea robin), and a perfectly good substitute for this is the blue-mouth (actually a relation of the true rascasse), a fish that is common in shallow, inshore UK waters, but, in our experience, never makes it to market. Goode (1887) regarded the sea scorpion as having no commercial value other than as bait, but in his *Fish Cookery*, James Beard describes sculpin (as it is known in the US) as 'an excellent food fish'; in Greenland, the sea scorpion is regarded as a delicacy, where it is called *kanajok* and cooked like cod. Even better than the sea scorpion is the weever fish, with its delicious, firm flesh. Again, you never see it in fish shops.

Then there is the lamprey, an eel-like creature with suckers in place of jaws that looks like a monster from the cover of a trashy sci-fi paperback. And all over the world there is the catfish, esteemed in Asia and in the Cajun cuisine of the southern states of America, but dismissed by many in the UK.

We also include a few fish that aren't so much ugly as for some reason uncool. Such fish are overlooked perhaps because they have 'grander' cousins. Megrim (or whiff) is related to turbot and brill, and while it's true it lacks the fine texture of these fish, it is a cheap and flavoursome alternative. We believe the fact that the vast majority of the huge amount of megrim landed in Cornwall is sold to Spanish fish dealers is indicative of something: Spanish consumers know their fish. The black sea bream bears no visual comparison to its classy, gilded Mediterranean counterpart the gilt-head bream, known in France as *daurade* and Greece as *tsipoúra*, but grilled over charcoal we defy you to tell the two apart. One bream-like fish found in Atlantic waters – Lagadon rhomboides, dubbed 'sailor's choice' in Goode's book, and similar to the sheepshead (with its strangely human teeth) – is particularly delicious. Humble dabs, flukes and flounders, which are abundant, tend to be under-rated because they are compared to Dover sole. The pompano is hardly a beauty, but it is sensational cooked in butter. Ray's bream – eaten the world over as pomfret – is also relatively common in Atlantic waters, but is ignored by most people in the UK. Ironically enough, if you are looking for Ray's bream in Britain, you're best off looking in an Indian or South-East Asian shop where you'll be able to buy it imported from China, India or Pakistan. Go figure.

Eat ugly fish!

Gills, gills, gills

American ichthyologist George Brown Goode writes of the wolf-fish, or sea catfish:

> It is impossible to imagine a more voracious-looking animal... with its massive head, and long, sinuous, muscular body, its long rayed fins and its vise-like [sic.] jaws armed with great pavements of teeth, those in front, long, strong pointed like those of a tiger, closely studded, reinforced in the rear by others rounded and molar like adapted for crushing the objects which have been seized by the carved teeth in the front of the jaw...

During his relatively short life, Goode was something of a force of nature, managing to maintain a prodigious publishing output whilst working as the secretary of the Smithsonian Institution in Washington. Together with British zoologists Francis Day and Frank Buckland, he laid the foundations of modern day ichthyology, that branch of zoology devoted to the study of fish. For more details of Buckland's diverse interests see page 221. Goode's 1887 *American Fishes: a Popular Treatise upon the Game and Food Fishes of North America with Especial Reference to Habits and Methods of Capture* may not have won the 1887-catchiest-title-prize, but it is most certainly a masterpiece of scholarly excellence. It is also, due to the miracle of the World Wide Web, available to download free in its entirety.

Building on the work of nineteenth-century pioneers, no one did more in the twentieth and early twenty-first century to promote, popularise and disseminate knowledge of fish and fish cookery than Alan Davidson. To anyone with a serious interest in fish, wherever they come from, we recommend unreservedly his excellent series of books: *North Atlantic Seafood*, *Mediterranean Seafood* and *Seafood of South-East Asia*. As well as being utterly comprehensive, they are written with great erudition and no small amount of wit. Mr Davidson's love for fish and seafood leaps off every page: no cook's home is complete without these books.

So what of Goode's wolf-fish? Well, it is an amazing creature, which, thanks to a natural anti-freeze it produces, can survive in icy waters. It also has a 'lockable' jaw, which will continue to bite down on objects placed in its mouth even when the head has been severed from the body. (If you don't believe us, you can check it out on YouTube.) The powerful jaws and 'great pavements' of teeth that Goode describes mean it is well equipped to crush and consume crabs, sea urchins and even whelks. If you want to know how powerful the jaws and teeth must be, try biting on a whelk shell next time you see one (actually, don't). The (wholly justified) Icelandic name for the wolf-fish is *steinbítur*: stone biter.

The wolf-fish is, in fact, very good to eat, and thrives in certain areas of the North Atlantic. But it is a seriously ugly fish. The Canadian government website 'Agriculture and Agri-Food Canada' translates it into French as *loup de mer* (European sea bass) rather than the correct *loup marin*. Anything to do with its ugliness, we wonder? Stocks, however, are low in places and before you even consider eating it, make sure you know the provenance of the specimen you are being offered (the New England coast, for example, is one of the places where wolf-fish stocks have been seriously depleted). The best parts – as with many fish – are the cheeks. In fact one of the main reasons for buying fish whole is that, especially with larger fish, you get a head that is full of flavour, gelatinous texture and meaty goodness. 'Penang fish-head curry' is a great delicacy in Malaysia.

The title of 'World's Ugliest Fish', however, must go to the blobfish. Indeed, the blobfish is the official mascot of the Ugly Animal Preservation Society. We didn't dare include an image of this hideous creature, but a Google search will reveal all. You have been warned.

The blobfish lives at extreme depths where the pressure is so great that the usual physiological systems fish have evolved for buoyancy do not work. It therefore manages to float because its body is a gelatinous, muscle-free mass, which is propelled by currents just above the sea bed. Until recently it was rarely caught, and hence barely seen by humans (no bad thing, perhaps). Unfortunately, the world's ugliest, most miserable looking fish now has reason to look the way it does. Modern super-deep-water fishing around Australia is driving it to extinction. We must learn.

And before you think that such horrors only lurk in the deep ocean... When in 2002 an angler in Maryland caught an 18-inch fish he didn't recognise, he did the right thing and took it to the Department of Natural Resources. At first the DNR were confused, then they identified the fish as a northern snakehead, a fish farmed in China to supply the huge demand for it as both a soup ingredient and a folk remedy.

Now the snakehead is a voracious carnivore, and it probably survived by feeding on native species such as bluegills and sunfish, so the DNR decided on a relatively non-invasive plan to isolate it within the pond in which it had been caught. That was until someone pointed out that the snakehead is unique in the fish world: not only can it breath air and survive out of water for up to four days, it can quite happily crawl around on land! The DNR had to act quickly before the snakehead made the short crawl 75 yards to a nearby river. Rumour has it that sharp shooters with rifles were placed along the pond edge, ready to shoot any snakeheads making a dash for freedom.

Earlier this year, the fish was spotted in a river in the east of England. The typically level headed response of the British tabloid media was to run an story under the headline 'Psycho Predator Is Sid Fishious', claiming that in China the fish is known to eat humans.

The reality is that while the snakehead is a voracious carnivore it has – as far as we know – never attacked a human. As well as that, while they can crawl on land, whoever suggested that they are able to breathe air was wrong.

They're just ugly fish.

Fin?

In general, sea fish are divided into two groups: coastal fish and oceanic fish. Coastal fish live in the area between the shoreline and the edge of the continental shelf, rarely at depths greater than 200 metres; oceanic fish, on the other hand, live beyond the continental shelf, some at unfathomable depths. In practice, and since there is a notable absence of border control, many species live between the two zones.

A further division is made between pelagic fish, those fish that live neither close to the surface of the water, nor to the bottom, and demersal fish, which live near the sea bed (those that live on or under the sea bed are known as 'benthic'). Some examples of coastal pelagic fish typically found in European waters are sardine, herring and mackerel. Coastal demersal fish, such as sole, turbot and plaice, are negatively buoyant and spend their lives on the ocean floor. Oceanic pelagic fish include tuna, marlin and swordfish. Oceanic demersal fish include the rat-tail (or 'hoki') and the hag-fish, discussed below.

The depths at which various fish live is a complex matter dependent on, rather obviously, whether they are pelagic or demersal, but also whether they are coastal or oceanic. Some bottom-dwelling demersal fish such as flounders live in extremely shallow coastal waters; in many parts of the world, you can paddle below knee-height and watch small dabs and flounders fanning sand on their backs near your feet in an effort not to be seen. The North Atlantic cod, while strictly speaking a demersal fish, is rarely found below 200 metres (which, in the great marine scheme of things, is not particularly deep). Indeed, most of the fish species traditionally fished commercially, whether they be pelagic or demersal, exist in the epipelagic, or sunlit, zone of the sea: the area that extends from the surface of the water to a depth of 200 metres.

It's interesting food for thought that this area is also called the 'surface' zone. In the world of recreational diving, any dive below thirty metres is referred to as a 'deep sea' dive. Bear in mind also that 75 per cent of the total volume of seawater in the world exists below a depth of 1000 metres, and a high percentage of that exists below a mean depth of 8000 metres. There's a whole world down there, and we know very little about it.

Notice, however, that while we know next-to-nothing about the world at these depths, that doesn't stop us taking horrendous liberties with it. It's a little known fact about the Apollo 13 – 'Houston... we have a problem...' – mission that a radioactive generator, originally destined to stay on the moon with the Lunar Excursion Module, was abandoned over the south-west Pacific. The 4 kilos of plutonium it contained is currently languishing somewhere between 6000 and 9000 metres down in the Tonga trench. It will remain radioactive for thousands of years.

Many oceanic pelagic fish exist in the bathypelagic zone, the undersea zone that begins about 500 metres below the surface, extending to a depth of 4000 metres. For many of the seas and oceans of the earth, the bathypelagic zone is as deep as it gets. There is little or no sunlight at these depths, and as such it is also known also as the 'midnight' zone. The water pressure is unimaginable, around 5800 pounds per square inch (humans, if they are lucky, can withstand about 50), it is extremely cold and there is little oxygen. The fish that exist at these depths have specially-adapted metabolisms to survive. They tend not to be choosy about what they eat since, unless you happen to be the size of a sperm whale, swimming around and searching for food is simply not an option. On the whole, then, bathypelagic fish simply lie still and wait for food to come along. The anglerfish, which is not only both pelagic and benthic, but actually inhabits a range of different depths (and seems to get uglier the deeper it goes) attracts food with its rod-like bioluminescent lure, hence the name 'angler'.

With dwindling fish stocks at less extreme depths, the fishing industry increasingly targets the bathypelagic zone. Many of the demersal fish that live here are eel-like in appearance: take the pacific hag-fish, for example, which coats itself in a slime made of rotting matter found on the seabed, rendering it inedible to other species; or the gulper eel, which possesses a mouth so totally out of proportion with the rest of its body that it can swallow prey much, much larger than itself.

According to a recent study, details of which have been posted by the journal *Science*, it has been discovered that the huge number of tiny mesopelagic fish that migrate daily to shallow waters in order to feed – there is little to no vegetation at the depths they inhabit – make a low frequency hum, about six decibels louder than background noise. In doing so, they are inadvertently sounding their own dinner bell.

And by 'their own dinner bell' we do not mean their own dinner.

They're dinner.

Gastronomically speaking, one of the most interesting fish found at these depths is the rat-tail, or grenadier. The grenadier, as it happens, is a delicious fish to eat, and it enjoyed a deal of popularity in the 1990s when it was marketed as 'hoki' (it is still found sometimes as Pacific 'hake' – the depths that fish marketing teams plumb are as great as those mined by industrial trawlers). In the 1979 edition of *North Atlantic Seafood*, Alan Davidson advises that rat-tails have 'quite a good texture and flavour' and that 'they constitute a considerable resource which is likely to be exploited more fully in the future'. With a degree of prescience, however, he adds that 'their growth rate is so slow that they might not withstand really heavy exploitation'. As with so many oceanic demersal fish, its longevity, along with its slow growth rate, make the rat-tail entirely the wrong kind of fish to be targeting.

And as we will also see, deep-sea fishing (so called 'bottom trawling') doesn't just target fish that are slow growing and long-lived – in other words utterly the wrong fish to be going for in the first place – but also causes absolute devastation to the sea bed itself, disrupting and in some cases destroying an already fragile eco-system.

In the March 2012 edition of *Marine Policy*, it was reported that:

> The combination of very low target population productivity, nonselective fishing gear, economics that favour population liquidation and a very weak regulatory regime makes deep-sea fisheries unsustainable with very few exceptions. Rather, deep-sea fisheries more closely resemble mining operations that serially eliminate fishable populations and move on.

> Instead of mining fish from the least-suitable places on Earth, an ecologically and economically preferable strategy would be rebuilding and sustainably fishing resilient populations in the most suitable places, namely shallower and more productive marine ecosystems that are closer to markets.

The orange roughey is another deep-sea demersal fish that was 'mined' for a sustained period between the 1970s, when it was first discovered, and the early twenty-first century. By 2010 the Australian authorities had officially declared the fish endangered and it is now on the Greenpeace 'red' list, the list of fish recognised as being sourced from entirely unsustainable fisheries.

You see, eating ugly fish is only one part of the solution. Imagine a world in which this book sells so widely (yes, imagine...) that it causes the demand, and hence the market for the gurnard or sea robin to expand hugely. The fish-consuming population of the Western world, tired after years of dining on boring red snapper or sea bass, simply can't get enough of the gurnard's firm, crustacean-enriched flesh.

The problem then is that the market drives fishermen to target the poor gurnard at the expense of other fish. What we need to establish is a balance,

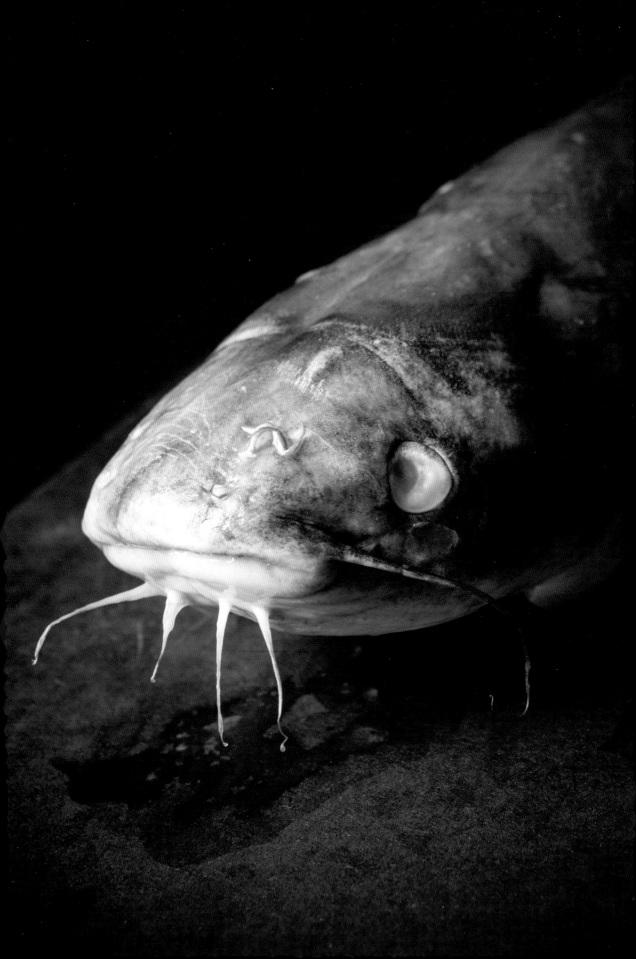

and that can only be achieved through a thorough understanding of the situation as it stands and how it is likely to unfold. Sustainability is a highly complex issue, a function of where the fish have been caught, how they have been caught and the complex system of quotas that have been put in place to regulate stocks.

Take, as just one example, the cod: the name 'cod' actually refers to a range of several, inter-related species of demersal (sometimes, semi-pelagic) fish – belonging to the family *gadidae* – that live in a wide range of habitats all around the world. The species includes the Pacific cod, the black cod (which thrives around New Zealand and Australia), the Atlantic cod and Greenland cod, as well as the haddock, hake, ling and pollack, all caught in British waters. Now if you have ever spent your summers next to a fjord in the far north of Norway, or live on the south coast of the UK, then the occasional cod caught with a rod and line (or even a small net) is perfectly sustainable. Indeed, catching fish singly in this manner (and not being wasteful and enjoying the whole fish) won't dent fish populations.

However, modern, industrial fishing is an entirely different kettle of... well, you know what we mean. The nets that the largest commercial 'bottom trawlers' drag along the sea bed are so big that some of them could happily accommodate a Boeing 747 jumbo jet. And while it was once thought that 'tilling' the seabed in this manner actually promoted productivity (in a manner analogous to ploughing a field), we now know it does immeasurable harm to the marine ecology. One study estimates that for every kilo of fish caught in a beam trawl, a form of bottom trawling that literally removes the surface of the seabed, 16 kg of marine life – including starfish and other echinoderms are killed.

'But humans don't eat starfish', we hear you cry. No, but fish do.

And industrial fishing boats are capable of catching truly incomprehensibly large numbers of fish. In the late 1950s, when cod were still caught by traditional methods (from small boats, with small nets) the annual Canadian cod catch amounted to 250,000 tons. By the late 1960s that figure had risen to 800,000 tons, and by the early 1990s, the cod were all but gone. Stocks may never recover.

If you live on the west coast of the US, by contrast, Pacific cod is a perfectly acceptable choice, but only if it is caught using a 'long-line', a length of line hung from a boat with baited hooks placed at equal intervals. It was recently estimated that a single bottom trawler would have the same impact on marine ecosystems as up to up to 1700 long-liners. As a result of strict quota systems, levels of North Sea cod appear to be recovering, but as a result many fish that are regarded 'by-catch' (including immature examples of the targeted fish) are dumped back into the sea, most of them dead. Between 1995 and 2000 it was estimated that 61 per cent of the total cod catch was discarded.

The Marine Conservation Society provides a free sustainable fish guide in the UK (the Monterey Bay Aquarium in the US and The Australian Marine Conservation Society do the same). Armed with one of these, you have no excuse for buying unsustainable fish wherever you are.

First take your fish

THE WHOLE FISH

Many people are nervous about buying whole fish, preferring as they do the neatly-shaped fillets known in the trade as 'bricks'. Did you know that, before they too became endangered, the majority of the entire Canadian catch of redfish (or ocean perch) used to be processed and then released into the US retail market as frozen fillets? How many litres of delicious soup, stew or fish-head curry are simply thrown away with the heads and carcasses? Where is the sense in our not consuming such ingredients? This is a recurring theme. Why do so many people insist on food products that bear absolutely no resemblance to their natural state? We want to challenge shoppers to think more about the relationship between the frozen fish fillet they have bought and the beautiful creature it originated from, to remind them of a time when buying a fish was precisely that, and not picking up a single boneless fillet from the freezer-cabinet.

And when you buy a whole fish, there is of course no requirement that you have the skills to gut, fillet and skin it: your fishmonger will do everything for you (and if s/he doesn't, then don't change your purchase, change your fishmonger). Besides which, we suspect that the real reason people find fish-filleting difficult is not some innate lack of ability, but rather the lack of a sharp knife. Invest in a decent knife and a decent sharpener: you will not regret it.

So, where possible, buy whole fish, and rise to the challenge of eating the whole beast and, in doing so, wasting nothing.

YES, BUT IS IT FRESH?

> Our habits of merchandising, of buying, and of living unhappily preclude, for the most part, the possibility of a fish's leaping directly from its habitat into the frying pan – and to the extent to which this is true the subtlest and most important part of fresh [...] fish cookery is lost to us.
>
> Richard Olney, *Simple French Food*, 1975

How to Tell if a Fish is Fresh

Your sense of smell is probably the one you should trust most. But use your other senses too. Look at the eyes: they should stand out, as if they're looking back at you. If they are sunken, that is a bad sign. Also, the gills of really fresh fish are bright red and almost shiny: if they are grey and dry, don't buy. Where possible, also use your fingers. If you prod a fish on a slab and your finger leaves an indentation, then that is not a good sign either: fresh fish is firm to the touch, not soft. And finally, fish that is fresh also has a covering of natural slime: it should feel moist not dry.

We're convinced that many people who say they don't like fish have simply never tasted fresh fish. That 'fishy' smell that people object to is not the smell of fish at all. Rather it's the smell and taste of fish that is beginning to spoil. Fresh fish smell of the sea. They smell salty.

Fairly obviously, then, it makes sense to be led by your nose in the purchase of fish. We realise that in many UK supermarkets fresh fish is sold, pre-filleted, in the same clear plastic packs that chicken breasts come in, and that you can't smell through a layer of plastic. But might this be the very reason such packs exist? Don't buy fish pre-packed in this way. Never buy fish pre-packed in this way. It is an insult to the fish, to the fisherman who has risked his life to catch it and to you, the discerning customer. Buy fish that is displayed openly, on ice, and if your local fishmonger objects to your smelling his/her produce, change your fishmonger. In many parts of the world, anyone selling fish and actively trying to prevent customers from smelling the fish would be run out of town (or, at the very least, go out of business very quickly). Why, in the Anglo-Saxon world, should things be any different?

In the main, fish spoil because of bacterial growth. The bacteria responsible for this spoiling live on the fish while it is alive, but once it dies they multiply quickly and attack the flesh: it's these bacteria that cause that fishy smell, and the disintegration of the flesh. Preserving fish successfully is achieved in the main by two methods. The first relies on temperature, for bacterial growth is greatly slowed if fish is kept in a cool environment. If it is kept well iced, the growth of bacteria on a dead fish is slowed down by about seven times. When frozen, bacterial growth is arrested completely, which is why frozen fish lasts so long. Salt also greatly reduces bacterial growth, so putting cleaned fish in a container of salt will preserve it well. (And if you put the container in your fridge it will last even longer.)

The second method revolves around depriving the bacteria of the water they need to survive and proliferate. The water content of a just landed fish is about 80 per cent. If you reduce that content to around 20 per cent, the bacteria simply die and the fish will last indefinitely. If you do decide to try the salting route, though, be aware that once most of the water has been driven off, you will be left with a product that is very different to the fish in its natural state. *Bacalhau* – Portuguese salted and dried cod – requires at least a couple of days reconstituting in fresh water, and then cooking like fresh cod. Other preparations are more forgiving: herring fillets that have been salted for a week are delicious simply rinsed well and eaten raw with rye bread, sour cream and onion.

RECIPES

All recipes serve 4 unless otherwise noted.

FISH SOUPS AND FISH STEWS

If ever there was a set of core techniques worth learning, it is those that turn whole fish into soups and stews. These dishes are simply delicious and among our favourite things to cook and eat (well, for one of us, our absolute favourite thing to cook and eat). Happily, whether a dish is a soup or a stew, the same core techniques – indeed the same ingredients – are used. From learning these core techniques it follows that you will able to cook a huge range of dishes.

But what is the difference between a soup and a stew? There are people who suggest that stews are thickened and soups are not. We disagree. We have eaten dishes that are undoubtedly 'soups' but which have been thickened with egg yolks, or cream. Others suggest that, in general, stews are cooked for longer than soups. Again, we disagree. In the case of fish, this is certainly not true. While beef and veal stews are happy to bubble away for hours and hours on end, fish stews and fish soups generally should not be cooked for longer than about 40 minutes. With some fish any longer than this and the bones will give your dish an unwanted bitterness. Indeed, we rarely leave fish bones bubbling in liquid longer than 25 minutes.

Pretty much the only difference we've managed to establish between a fish soup and a fish stew is the relation between the quantity of solids and the quantity of liquid in the finished dish. In general, a soup tends to be mostly, or, indeed, completely, liquid (a consommé, after all, is a kind of soup). A stew, by contrast, contains more solids in relation to the cooking liquid, whether in the form of fish, vegetables, rice, pasta, or other.

It's up to you, of course. But whatever you decide to call the dish you have cooked, also bear in mind that while a thick soup is sometimes highly desirable, a thin stew never is.

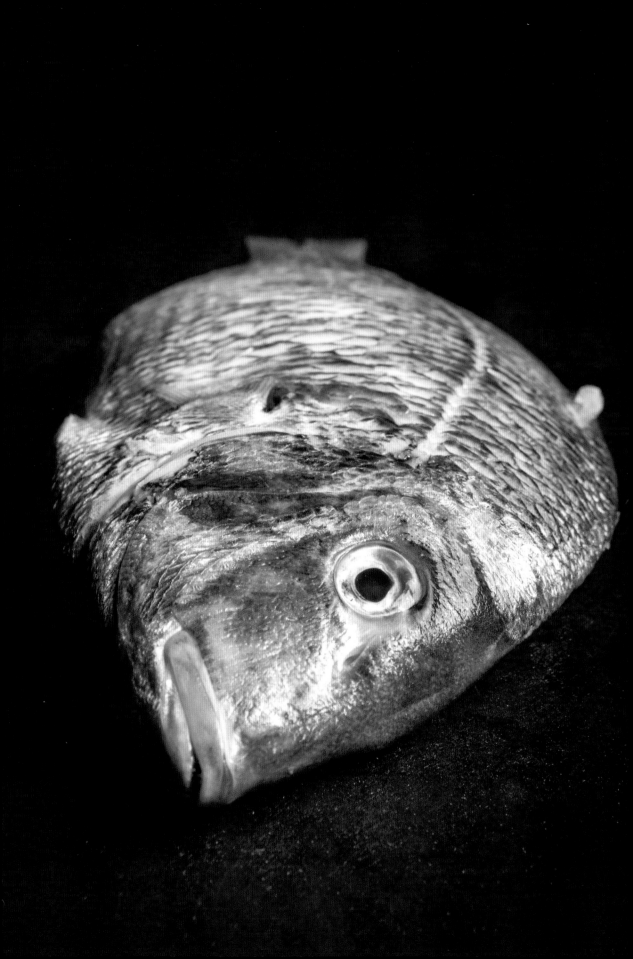

The Basics

1kg whole fish (filleted or not)

aromatics

liquid

The fish, of course, will vary. The aromatics will vary too. As you'll see in the recipes below, those in a Norman Marmite Dieppoise are very different to those in a Greek Kakaviá; those in Malaysian fish Laksa are different to those in a Thai fish curry. The liquid also will depend on the recipe. In Europe, wine is often, but not always used. South-East Asian soups and stews often call for coconut milk. Many fish soups/stews around the world actually incorporate a good splash of local seawater for seasoning. (We recommend exercising caution on this point.)

In very simple terms, the core technique(s) involved in preparing fish soups and stews include the following stages:

1. Cook the aromatics and flavourings in oil.

2. Add the bones of the fish, and sometimes a head or two (notice with some dishes, you might want to add whole fish, but the cooking time will reduce).

3. Add an appropriate liquid, typically water, wine or stock.

It's also very common for these first three stages to be condensed into one: put everything in a capacious pot.

4. Simmer gently for 30-40 minutes.

5. Strain out the bones and heads.

6. Return the stock to the pan.

7. If you cooked the stock without the fillets, add these and cook gently until they are cooked through.

8. Finish or thicken the dish in whatever way you have decided.

Pretty much every recipe for fish soup or stew we give below is an elaboration on these basic stages. It really is that simple. (And you would be perfectly justified in seeing parallels between these core techniques and those that lie behind the cooking of meat soups/stews – whilst recognising, of course, crucial differences in the timing of each.)

Kakaviá

When most people think of Mediterranean fish soup/stew, they think of the authentic Bouillabaisse de Marseille. Bouillabaisse is delicious, but please bear in mind that it has transcended its position as a mere 'dish' and is now the stuff of culinary folklore (or even, according to Richard Olney, 'philosophy'). The presentation of Bouillabaisse nowadays in restaurants in the South of France is typically as much about theatre as it is about gastronomy, what with schools of identically besuited waiting staff flitting from table to table with spoons and fish slices, skinning and deboning cooked fish at a rate of knots. And it is because of this, as much as it is because of the price of Mediterranean fish, that *bouillabaisse* for four – and just Bouillabaisse – could easily set you back €300 (€150-€200 more if you want your Bouillabaisse bolstered with a *langouste* or two! It's good. But is it really that good?

We tend to prefer a humble fisherman's dish of the kind from which *bouillabaisse* almost certainly evolved. Our friend, Greek poet Patricia Kolaiti, cooked us her Kakaviá out of season in her home in Aegina, Greece and, in doing so, gave us a lesson in harmony and simplicity. This is our version of her dish.

1kg of small rockfish (the Greeks call these *petrósparo*),
gutted and seasoned with salt

500g chopped onions

500g chopped tomatoes

250ml olive oil

2 lemons

bread

garlic

1. Put the onion, tomatoes, olive oil and salt in a deep pot.

2. Cover with water, bring to the boil and cook steadily for 40 minutes.

3. Add the fish and cook for 15 minutes more, maintaining the same steady boil.

4. Remove the fish, put onto slices of toast rubbed with garlic and place in a serving bowl.

5. Add a generous quantity of lemon to the liquid in the pot, and pour it over the fish and toast.

There are equivalents to the Greek *petrósparo* in English waters. They are, no doubt, slightly different in character – after all, they enjoy a different diet, and are exposed to far less sunlight – but we doubt this renders them entirely without culinary value. There are probably a number of reasons why such fish never come to market. Most obviously, of course, there is no demand (and there is a range of reasons for this – they're ugly, bony, and so on). But also, it's probably true that catching fish in the required quantities around the rocky shorelines of, say, Devon and Cornwall, would be no easy matter. In theory, however, there is no reason why British rockfish soup should not be up there with the very best. We certainly have the fish – the various gobies, blue-mouths and other sea-scorpions, weever fish, blennies, clingfish, rockling and the like.

Who will be the first celebrity chef to tap into this huge potential, we wonder?

Or will someone read this recipe and rise to the challenge of championing British ugly fish soup?

Bourride

Bourride, the dish that is sometimes described as the Languedoc version of bouillabaisse, is so different to its Provençal cousin that the two dishes are barely comparable. Happily, however, the differences mean that it is much easier to recreate outside the South of France than its Marseillaise counterpart. While people do wax lyrical about it, it has not quite achieved the folklore status of bouillabaisse, since the key to success is not the rockfish of Marseille (nor the theatrical way in which it is served) but, rather, that garlicky confection aioli.

This is our version. For an absolutely authentic recipe, consult your copy of *French Provincial Cooking* by Elizabeth David. You don't have one? You need one. Get your hands on one of the best books on food ever written.

> 1kg of one or two varieties of firm white fish – anglerfish, sea bass, John Dory, brill, gurnard (filleted, but with the head and the bones)
> 2 leeks, white and light green parts only, thinly sliced
> small bunch of parsley, roughly chopped
> (and a few more finely-chopped leaves for garnish)
> a slice of lemon
> a quantity of aioli made from 2 egg yolks and 500ml olive oil (see page 48)
> sea salt

1. Put the sliced leek, chopped parsley and lemon in a large pot.

2. Add the bones of the fish and cover with about 750ml of water.

3. Simmer for half an hour or so and strain. Discard the solids and return the stock to a clean pan.

4. Season your fish fillets and poach them in the stock until they are just cooked.

The next bit is incredibly easy (if we can do it, it must be) but do take care; you are, effectively, thinning with warm liquid an already emulsified mixture of egg yolks and oil.

5. Into your large bowl of thick, gloriously golden aioli slowly pour – whisking all the time – about 200ml of the stock in which the fish has been cooked; the sticky garlic mayonnaise will turn the texture of thick double cream.

6. Now add another 200ml of stock to the aioli; it will become a little thinner, but still of double cream thickness.

7. Place the cooked fish into a shallow serving bowl.

8. Again whisking all the time, turn the contents of your bowl of aioli into the liquid in the pan and – while being careful not to let the mixture boil – warm through thoroughly; once mixed together with the aioli mixture the sauce will now have the texture of single cream.

9. Garnish with parsley and serve with steamed potatoes or slices of bread fried in olive oil.

More aioli to put on the fried bread or mash with the potatoes is wonderful, but don't plan on kissing anyone that night who has not shared your Bourride with you.

Or, alternatively, don't bother cooking Bourride for people you wouldn't happily kiss.

Arroz a Banda

Sometimes you will have bought, say, a whole filleted gurnard and fried the fillets (as we suggested at the beginning of this chapter). If you freeze the head and the bones of each fish you buy, you will quickly have an amount worth using. This Spanish delicacy is a wonderful way of using them, and we include it immediately after our recipe for Bourride because it too is delicious served with aioli.

250g long grain rice
500ml fish stock
(simply follow stages 1-3 of the Bourride recipe and reduce accordingly)
half a teaspoon of saffron strands, toasted very gently in a dry pan

1. Place the rice, stock and saffron strands in a large pan.

2. Bring to the boil and simmer gently until the liquid has all but disappeared and the rice is almost cooked.

3. Remove from the heat, cover and leave to rest for 5 minutes.

4. Serve with aioli.

Unexpectedly delicious.

Variation on a Chaudrée

> A Chaudrée is a marvellous fish soup which they make in Charentes, but a real Chaudrée requires the fish of the district and special shellfish. Since I have neither the one nor the other I shall make my own version of Chaudrée. For six people I shall buy a good 3lbs of various kinds. The less elegant sorts of fish such as conger eel, rock salmon and the heads, of gurnards, if you can get them, will all be useful.

Edouard de Pomiane, *Cooking with Pomiane*, 1976

We both prefer reading books about food than we do 'cookbooks' per se. We've tried to write this volume as an antidote to the flick-through, 'cherry tomatoes in summer sunlight' genre of cookbook, which are intended for the sitting room table, not the kitchen (or even the bedside table). Perhaps we were lucky, but for whatever reason we discovered writers such as Elizabeth David and Edouard de Pomiane fairly early on in our culinary explorations. Elizabeth David called de Pomiane's writing 'the best kind of cookery writing' and who are we to disagree? He was certainly opinionated and sometimes dismissive of some of the classics of haute cuisine.

He prefaces his recipe for *Homard à l'Americaine* as follows:

> This is a celebrated dish, but it offends a basic principle of taste. The sauce, which is too highly spiced and too rich in tomato and brandy, kills the delicate flavour of the lobster. With this reservation in mind one can eat it from time to time.

De Pomiane's recipe for Chaudrée is typical of his writing. It is playful and witty, but at the same time full of knowledge and imbued with a strong sense of what are the right and proper ways to prepare and serve food. This recipe is for six people.

1.5kg mixed huss (rock salmon), conger eel and gurnard
(we doubt you'd find a fishmonger willing to sell you a gurnard head –
so buy the whole thing)
2 bottles of dry white wine (yes, we baulked a little at first too)

2 cloves of garlic

4 shallots

pinch of nutmeg

2 bay leaves

2 eggs

125g double cream

125g butter

salt and freshly-ground black pepper

1. Pour all the wine into a large pan and place over a high heat.

2. Add the gurnard head and bones to the wine; add the finely chopped garlic and shallots, a turn or two of black pepper, a pinch of nutmeg and the 2 bay leaves.

3. Once the wine has come to the boil, turn the heat down and simmer for 30-40 minutes, skimming when you need to; strain.

4. Having divided the fish into pieces 'about as big as an egg' (who other than de Pomiane would have thought to give such a simple, but such a perfect guide to portioning?) place them in the simmering stock and cook for 20 minutes or so, until the fish is nicely cooked.

5. Remove the fish from the pan and keep warm in a low oven.

6. In a soup tureen (or whatever bowl you plan to bring the soup to the table in), beat the eggs and cream together and set to one side for a moment.

7. Whisk the butter slowly into the bouillon over a low heat and when it is all amalgamated add it to the serving bowl or tureen; it will turn white and smell utterly delicious.

8. Add the fish and serve the soup in large bowls.

De Pomiane finishes his recipe as follows:

> Into the glasses I pour Chavignol, so chilled that there is a delicate mist on the glasses. I watch the faces of my guests. I am happy. They are filled with contentment.

Marmite Dieppoise

If ever there were an indicator of the vanishingly vast difference between the food cultures of northern France and southern England it is to be found at either end of the four-hour ferry trip between Newhaven, East Sussex and Dieppe, France. Dieppe has countless fresh fish shops, Newhaven has two or three at most; Dieppe has hundreds of top, top quality fish restaurants, Newhaven has none. Not one. Yes, there are a few nice Indian places, a couple of Italian trattoria and several pubs; but is there a single fish restaurant? No.

It is claimed that Marmite Dieppoise was 'invented' in the 1960s by a Mme Maurice, the cook in a Dieppe restaurant called, oddly enough, La Marmite Dieppoise. The restaurant is still there in Rue Saint-Jean and still serves this dish. (Though neither of us has been there for some time.) The recipe is particularly worthy of inclusion because, unlike fish dishes from the South of France, we have all the ingredients for it available locally in the UK. As a point of interest, one UK website claiming to have the actual recipe cooked at the restaurant in question claims it is made with burbot, a freshwater fish. We think it is highly unlikely a chef in Dieppe would look inland for a freshwater variety to cook with and suspect in this instance it is a mistranslation of *barbue*, the French word for brill. (For another example of the problems inherent in translating ingredients see our recipe for eel-pout in red wine below.)

On the question of whether Mme Maurice 'invented' the dish we remain agnostic. She no doubt played a huge role in popularising it among tourists and travellers to Dieppe, but as a recipe it's really just an application of the kind of core techniques central to making a Sole Dieppoise (Dover sole with mussels and prawns in a cream sauce) to a range of different fish at the same time.

It's a very convivial dish, however, and truly delicious. The following recipe is for eight people.

4kg whole fish – flounder, lemon sole, John Dory, gurnard, pollack (or sustainable cod); if you're feeling flush, you can include some prime fish too – brill and Dover sole (but if you've got your hands on 8 plump Dover sole, don't make *Marmite* – make *Sole* Dieppoise...)

500g of small, shell-on prawns (try not to buy peeled prawns; all the flavour is in the shells – shell them yourself and use the shells in the stock)

1kg live mussels in shells

250ml dry white wine

100g unsalted Normandy butter (let's do this properly)

2 onions, chopped

2 sticks of celery, chopped (and some of the leaves too)

2 leeks, chopped

1 fennel bulb, chopped

salt and freshly-ground black pepper

40g flour

250ml double cream

a pinch of cayenne pepper and/or curry powder

parsley leaves, chopped

1. Ask your fishmonger to fillet the fish (and don't forget to keep the heads and bones).

2. Cover the heads and bones of the fish, and the shells of the prawns, with about 1.5 litres of water; bring to the boil and simmer for 25 minutes. Drain and reserve the liquid.

3. While the stock is bubbling, pour the wine into another large pot, add the mussels, cover with the heaviest lid you have, and place over a high heat for about 5 minutes, shaking the pan occasionally. Remove the lid, and drain off the mussels reserving the liquid; remove the top shell of the mussels and put them to one side with the peeled prawns.

4. Heat 50g butter in the largest pot you have and add the chopped vegetables; they must not brown, but they should get good and soft. If they do begin to brown, the best way to prevent further overheating is to add a little stock.

5. Add the fish stock, bring to a very gentle simmer and add the pieces of fish; the gurnard and pollack will take longer than the sole or flounder, so use your judgement. The fish will take no longer than 7-8 minutes to cook; when it is cooked, remove and set to one side covered with a tea towel.

6. Find the most beautiful (yet practical) serving bowl you have, and let it warm in the oven.

7. Strain the reserved mussel cooking liquid into the pot with the stock, and give the pot in which you cooked your mussels a little rinse.

8. In the empty pot, heat the remaining butter and make a roux with the flour.

9. Once the roux is established, begin adding the stock slowly until you have a rich, velvety sauce; it shouldn't be too thin, but it doesn't want to be gloopy.

10. Now add the cream, cayenne pepper and curry powder; taste for salt – you may need a little, but the mussels will have given out plenty during their cooking time, so it's an idea to leave seasoning until the end.

11. Let it bubble away for 5 minutes. Don't worry about boiling double cream, it won't curdle, but will just reduce to an even richer consistency.

12. Remove the serving bowl from the oven and half fill it with the sauce. Add the fish, mussels and prawns, and then add the other half of the sauce; sprinkle with parsley and serve with steamed, peeled potatoes.

The cayenne pepper and curry powder may seem unlikely, but Dieppe has a long history of connections with the spice trade, so you should not be too surprised. If you want to, you can really go to town with this recipe. A dozen langoustines or scallops, or even a couple of lobsters do not seem out of place.

If you do happen to have eight Dover sole (they're not that ugly, but the price is hideous...), then follow the above recipe but:

1. Have the fish skinned but left on the bone.

2. Make the stock with vegetables, fish skins, prawn shells and mussel stock. Strain and reduce by half.

3. Bake the sole in the oven with a little white wine and stock.

4. Follows stages 8-11 above, but add neither cayenne nor curry powder; a hint of lemon juice is all you'll need.

5. Serve the sole on individual plates, with the sauce poured round and mussels and prawns tumbled over them.

Malaysian Fish Laksa

'Nyonya' cuisine is the name given to the style of cooking brought to Malaysia, Indonesia and Singapore by Chinese migrants. Laksa is a noodle soup thickened with coconut milk, rather than a stew, and the recipe also works well with fish heads.

1kg whole fish – gurnard or pollack would be perfect
250g small, shell-on prawns
175g rice noodles
400ml can of coconut milk
100g beansprouts
light muscovado sugar (or palm sugar if you can get it)
sea salt

To make the laksa spice paste, combine the following ingredients in a food processor and blend to a fine consistency:

3 or 4 hot red chillies

25g dried shrimps (soak them in water for 20 minutes before using)

2 lemongrass stalks, outer leaves removed

2 cloves of garlic, finely chopped

30g piece of root ginger

25g cashew nuts

1 shallot, finely chopped

large pinch of ground coriander

large pinch of turmeric powder

a small glass of water

For the garnish:

1 cucumber, peeled, de-seeded and sliced thinly

3 spring onions, white and light green parts only, thinly sliced

coriander leaves, chopped

2 red chillies, thinly sliced

1. Ask your fishmonger to fillet the fish, and keep the heads and bones; cut the fillets into smallish pieces.

2. Cover the heads and bones of the fish, and the shells of the prawns, with about 1 litre of water; bring to the boil and simmer for 25 minutes; drain and reserve the liquid.

3. Heat some oil in a large pan and add the laksa spice paste; keep moving it around for 4-5 minutes and look for the moment that the spices begin to start separating from the oil; at this point add your fish stock and cook for 20 minutes or so.

4. In a separate pan, simmer the rice noodles in water until they are just cooked; drain and reserve.

5. Add the coconut milk to the fish stock and cook for 3 minutes; add the fish and cook for about 3 minutes more (how long the fish takes will depend on the size of the pieces); add the beansprouts and cook for one minute.

6. Season with salt and sugar.

7. To serve, place noodles in four soup bowls. Top with the pieces of fish and a generous quantity of the soup. Garnish with thinly sliced cucumber and spring onions, coriander leaf and finely sliced red chillies.

It's not particularly authentic to season 'Nyonya' food with fish sauce (*nam pla*). But (full disclosure) we often season our European dishes with the stuff, so go ahead and give it a try.

Nam Pla

We always have a bottle of Thai fish sauce in our fridge, and would suggest you do too. It's an essential ingredient for a wide range of South-East Asian dishes, and no Thai meal is complete without a small bowl of *prik nam pla* (fish sauce with chopped bird's eye chillies) on the table. But it also adds a nice umami kick to just about any fish dish, and many meat dishes too, particularly those containing lamb.

MISCELLANEOUS FISH DISHES (AND A MOLLUSC AND A LAGOMORPH)

Roast Fish with Tomatoes, Garlic and Potatoes (and bacon, if you like)

This is a hearty meal that adapts perfectly to its surroundings: it is equally at home as a warming supper or a light summer lunch. The idea is that the dish will form the centrepiece of a meal for four people; you therefore need a fish of around 1kg. If your fish is smaller than that (or if you have a thick steak from a larger fish), you may need to parboil your potatoes, since you want the fish and the potatoes to be cooked at the same time.

1kg fish (black bream, gurnard, red porgy, Ray's bream, sheepshead...)

2 onions, finely chopped

3 cloves garlic, finely chopped

100g of streaky bacon cut into lardons (optional)

3 large tomatoes (peeled and deseeded) – use a can of tomatoes (drained) if good ripe tomatoes are hard to find

1 glass white wine

50g butter

4 medium size potatoes, peeled and cut into 2cm dice

olive oil

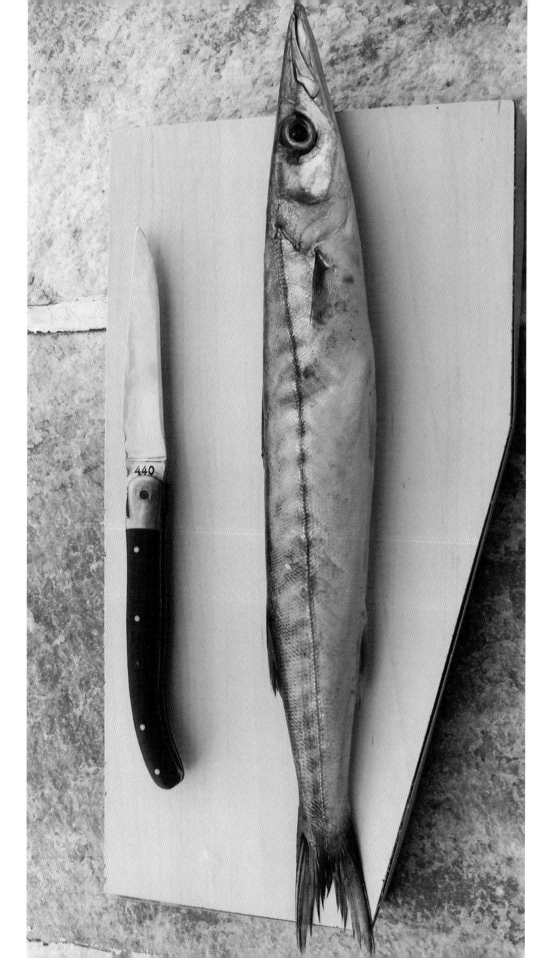

1. Pre-heat the oven to 200°C.

2. Sauté the onions and garlic in olive oil until soft (with the chopped bacon, if using).

3. Add the tomatoes and white wine and reduce to a thick, but not jammy consistency. (If it does get jammy, loosen with some water.)

4. Add the butter and leave the mixture to cool. (The cooling is important.)

5. Spread half the cooled mixture in an ovenproof pan that is large enough to hold the fish and the potatoes.

6. Slash the fish on each side and season inside and out with salt and freshly-ground black pepper (be generous).

7. Add the fish and potatoes to the pan.

8. Top with the remaining half of the sauce and toss with your fingers so that the fish and potatoes are well coloured and coated with the sauce (this is why the mixture needs to cool – the sauce needs to be evenly distributed and you can only really do this with fingers).

9. Add a generous quantity of olive oil and place in the hot oven.

10. Cook for 20 minutes to half an hour and then check. If it's all looking a little dry, add a small glass of water. Remember, though, that you're aiming to roast the contents of the pan, not braise them. The potatoes should be taking on a nice colour and the fish should have little scorch marks on the pectoral fins and extremities. Be bold.

11. Cook for another 20 minutes until the fish comes away from the bones where you made the slashes and the potatoes are crispy outside and soft and fluffy within.

Enjoy with a glass of wine, and don't ignore the head.

Megrim with Vermouth and Cream

As mentioned earlier, about 95 per cent of the Cornish megrim catch is sold to the Spanish wholesale business. We find megrim infinitely preferable to plaice and would encourage you to seek it out if you can. Megrim does have a tendency to be a little dry, and the creamy vermouth sauce works well to counteract that.

4 megrim, about 200g each – cleaned, but with heads on
125g unsalted butter
100ml Noilly Prat (or other dry vermouth)

125ml double cream

sea salt

lemon juice

1. Pre-heat the oven to 200°C.

2. Take an oven-proof tray or dish large enough to hold the four fish in a single layer. Smear the tray with the butter.

3. Season the megrim with salt on both sides and put in the tray.

4. Drizzle the vermouth over the fish (less is more, you may not need the full amount for 4 fish).

5. Bake in the oven for 10–12 minutes, until the fish is just cooked.

6. Pour the juice that has come off the fish into a small saucepan, bring to the boil, reduce by about a third and add the double cream. Heat until it thickens and add salt and lemon juice to taste.

7. Pour the creamy sauce over the fish and heat under a very hot grill until bubbling.

Enjoy with some nice bread and a bowl of fresh watercress (no salad dressing is necessary).

Eel-Pout in Red Wine

Madame Simone Prunier was a legendary London restaurateur. In her excellent *Fish Cookery Book*, first published in 1938, she includes four recipes for eel-pout, an under-used sea fish. Admittedly, Mme Prunier also includes over 180 preparations for sole, but this reflects the kind of 'high cookery' with which she was largely concerned.

We have found fish resembling eel-pout in the Mediterranean, but have not, thus far, come across it in fish shops in the UK. Fish cooked in red wine, however, is always a winner, and if you do happen to come across it (eel-pout is also known as muttonfish or ocean pout in the US), Mme Prunier's recipe is certainly worth trying.

The fish also provides a nice illustration of the complexities involved in reliably cross-referencing lesser-known fish between countries and across culinary cultures. To quote Alan Davidson, it is a veritable 'labyrinth'. In her recipe, Mme Prunier translates eel-pout into French as *lotte*, a word which is generally used in France to refer to anglerfish (Prunier translates anglerfish as *lotte-de-mer*). In many sources we have found, the French word *lotte* also refers to the burbot, a freshwater fish related to cod (from Latin *lota lota*) and, indeed, in her discussion of eel-pout Mme Prunier makes a great deal of the value of eel-pout liver, for which she provides a recipe. However, she surely means burbot liver, which was once highly prized. The residents of Walker, Minnesota hold an annual Eel-Pout Festival, and have done since 1979, but in Minnesota the word 'eel-pout' refers, you've guessed it, to burbot.

Despite that fact that in the sixteenth century burbot was so common that it was used as pig-feed, it is now thought to be extinct in the British Isles. In the 1960s *The Angling Times* offered a £100 reward to anyone catching one, a sum that remains unclaimed. The bottom line, then, is that if you do find eel-pout on sale in the UK, it is likely to really be eel-pout (which Alan Davidson translates into French as *loquette* – though, note, he does follow it with a question mark). But since it is not clear that Mme Prunier's recipe doesn't actually call for burbot, US readers might also want to try this recipe with that (and let us know how it turns out). We use anglerfish in our adaptation of her dish.

1kg of anglerfish tail on the bone

For the poaching liquor:

500ml of good red wine

sprig of thyme

bay leaf

clove of garlic, crushed

a glug of olive oil

sea salt

For the sauce:

2 or 3 shallots, finely chopped

150g unsalted butter

caster sugar

balsamic vinegar

1. Prepare the poaching liquor by adding to a shallow pan the red wine, thyme, bay leaf, crushed garlic, olive oil and salt.

2. Remove the anglerfish fillets from either side of the central bone (which, in the case of this fish, is cartilage) and add the bone to the liquor too.

3. Bring the poaching liquor to the boil, season the fish fillets well, and lay them in the liquor. Poach gently until just cooked (about 10 minutes).

4. In a separate pan, sauté the shallots gently in 100g of the butter; add a little sugar to get the caramelisation really going, then a generous splash of balsamic vinegar. (It will bubble and splutter as the liquid cooks off.)

5. Ladle about 200ml of the cooking liquor into the shallot and vinegar mixture; reduce by half.

6. Just before serving, add the remaining butter and shake the pan vigorously so it incorporates into the sauce.

Serve the fish on individual white plates, surrounded by the sauce. It is as utterly delicious as it is visually arresting.

Fillets of John Dory with Sauce 'Deauvillaise'

This is a delicious, typically under-stated recipe for John Dory from *French Provincial Cooking*. Elizabeth David was ahead of her time when it came to trying to make people think differently about ugly fish:

> [I]n some parts of France the St. Pierre is known as *l'horrible*, which seems rather unfair to the poor St. Pierre, for, while certainly no beauty, it has an expression of melancholy about its great head rather than anything savage or horrible.

2kg John Dory – this might seem a lot for four people,
but a single 500g John Dory will yield only around 150-175g of fillet;
make sure you keep the head and the bones; you can freeze
two of them since you'll only need two for the sauce

butter

breadcrumbs

For the sauce 'Deauvillaise':

butter

100g onion, finely sliced

head and bones of two John Dory (well rinsed)

125ml dry white wine or cider

250ml water

225ml double cream

1 teaspoon Dijon mustard

salt and freshly-ground black pepper

1. Melt some butter in a heavy-bottomed pan and cook the onion very gently; it must not brown.

2. While the onion slowly softens, make a small quantity of fish stock by adding two of the fish carcasses to a pan with the wine, the water and a little salt; if you have a small leek and a carrot, chop these and add them too; let it simmer gently for 20 minutes or so.

3. When the onion is very soft, push it through a sieve into a bowl.

4. Add a splash of the stock to the onion purée, the cream, mustard, salt and pepper and set to one side; all of this can be done well in advance, so this is a nice dish to cook for guests you want to spend time with.

5. About 10 minutes before you want to eat, turn on your grill to high.

6. Poach the fish gently in some of the stock that remains and when it is barely cooked, drain and place the fish in an oval gratin dish (or individual gratin dishes); top with the warmed sauce, sprinkle with a few breadcrumbs and a little butter and put them under the grill for between 2 and 3 minutes.

Elizabeth David suggests arranging little triangles of bread fried in butter around the edge of the gratin dish (or, if you have done separate dishes, around the edge of each dish). For many readers – particular those in the UK who associate fried bread with eggs, bacon and breakfast – this might seem entirely inappropriate. But trust Elizabeth David, a few slices of buttery fried bread is precisely what is needed to counteract the softness of the fish and the creamy mouth-feel of the sauce.

Fillets of black bream are also excellent served this way.

Cação Coentrada (Huss with Coriander 'Pesto')

Some of the recipes we have seen for this dish suggest that it is a soup, but when we've eaten it in Portugal it was very much fish with sauce (and served on a plate). Huss (or dogfish, or rock salmon, or rough-hound, or smooth-hound, or nurse-hound) is a fairly ugly beast. It's a species of shark.

4 huss steaks
100ml extra virgin olive oil
1 head of garlic, finely chopped
1 onion, finely chopped
a large bunch of coriander, finely chopped

500ml fish stock (made from the tail of the huss, or bones you have frozen)
30g plain flour
50ml wine vinegar
salt and freshly-ground black pepper

1. Warm 80ml of the olive oil in a large pan and slowly cook the garlic and onion until soft.

2. Add in all the coriander and pour on the fish stock; bring to the boil.

3. Add the slices of huss and poach for 5-10 minutes until they are cooked.

4. Remove the fish and keep warm.

5. Blend the sauce with a stick blender, or in a food processor.

6. Make a roux with the flour and the remaining olive oil and add the garlic-onion-coriander sauce slowly; it should be about the thickness of double cream.

7. Add salt, pepper and vinegar to taste (we doubt you'll want 50ml of vinegar, but you shouldn't be too shy).

8. Put the pieces of huss on 4 plates and pour on lots of sauce; serve with toasted bread.

Sakano-na-Ara (the bony parts)

It would be a mistake to think that the only use for fish heads and bones is to give flavour and body to stocks. On page 81 we provide a recipe for roast fish heads. Here is another recipe, courtesy of our colleagues Mrs Akiko Tsuda and Mr Norio Matsukuma, and is published in their hugely informative and enjoyable book *Recipes of Fukuoka* (2009). It makes use of the heads and bones of black bream, the flesh of which has been presented as sashimi. Either use the head and bones of two fish or – if you'd rather have a higher flesh-to-bone ratio – one whole fish. The dish also calls for burdock root, which we describe in our chapter **Ugly Veg**.

one 500g black bream, cleaned, or the heads and bones of 2 fish
200g burdock root
sugar snaps or mange-touts

A simmering liquid made of:

1.5 litres water
800ml sake

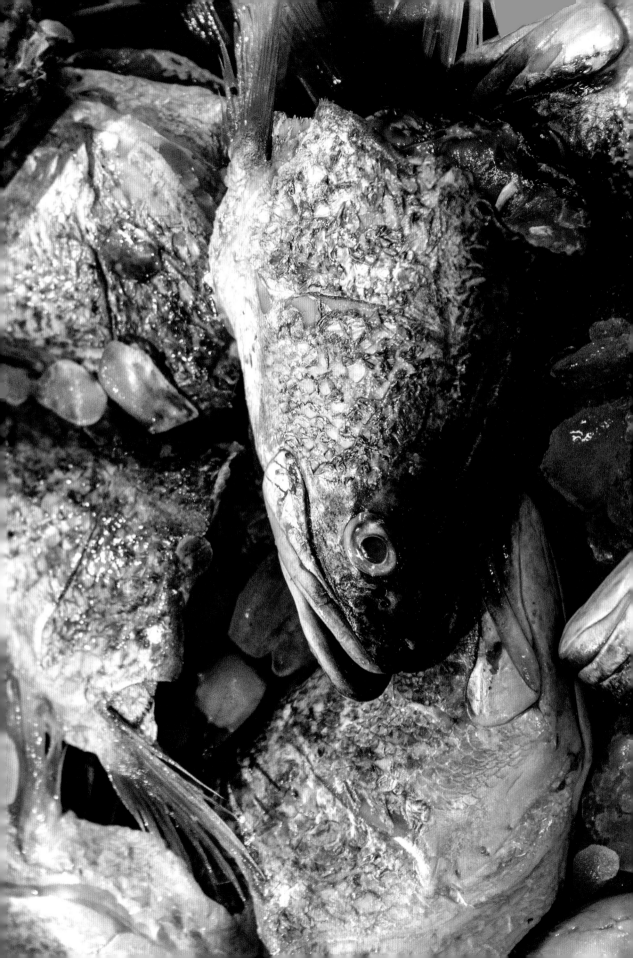

40g sugar

80ml mirin

800ml soy sauce – best to use the relatively cheap dark soy sauce available in Chinese supermarkets rather than an expensive one such as Kikkoman (which is our general preference)

1. If you're using one whole fish, cut off the head and tail (dispose of the gills), and slice the body in two lengthways and then across into three (giving you six pieces). If you're using the heads and bones of 2 fish, cut off the heads and tails and cut the spine into 3 pieces.

2. Prepare the burdock root as on page 191 and soak in acidulated water; blanch the sugar snaps or mange-touts.

3. Place the burdock in a pan, put the fish and/or bones on top and pour in the sake and the water; cover with a drop lid (a wooden lid which sits on the contents of the pan rather than the pan itself) and simmer. Alternatively, a cartouche would work.

4. When the eyeballs of the fish turn opaque, remove the lid, add the sugar and mirin and continue simmering until the liquid in the pan has reduced by about a third.

5. Add the soy sauce in small quantities and keep spooning the liquid over the fish and burdock; add the sugar snaps or mange-touts.

6. Place the fish and/or bones in a serving bowl and place the burdock and sugar snaps or mange-touts next to the fish. Cover with the stock, which smells utterly delicious.

Japanese food can be so delightfully clean tasting. Enjoy the broth and the vegetables. Slurp the flesh from the heads and bones (and enjoy the flesh too if you've used whole fish).

Arroz de Lampreia

Henry I, it is said, died from eating a 'surfeit of lampreys'. His physicians warned him constantly about the dangers of eating the fish, which always disagreed with him, but he just could not resist. The Latvians like their lampreys jellied, much as Londoners still enjoy jellied eel. The Spanish (well, Gallegos) and Portuguese make an excellent dish from lamprey, rice and lamprey blood. It is cooked in three stages: first the lamprey is cooked, then the rice and finally the lamprey and sauce are added to the rice and warmed through.

1kg of lamprey, cut into steaks
5 cloves of garlic, finely chopped
small bunch of parsley, finely chopped
500ml red wine
200ml lamprey blood
1 onion, chopped
250g long-grain rice
2 bay leaves
salt and freshly-ground black pepper

1. Place the lamprey steaks, the garlic, parsley, red wine and blood in a bowl; leave to marinate for 6 to 8 hours.

2. Heat the olive oil in a large pan and sauté the chopped onion slowly until soft.

3. Add the lamprey steaks to the onions and turn them over gently for 10 minutes or so; then add the wine and blood mixture. Continue to cook slowly until the lamprey is cooked. Season well.

4. Put the rice in a saucepan and add as much of the wine and blood sauce as you can without leaving the lamprey dry. (This is important because the final dish should have a similar liquid quality to the Arroz do Polvo on page 44.) Top up with water, season well and cook until the rice is just tender.

5. Add the lamprey and remaining sauce to the rice, mix well and serve nice and hot.

The finished dish should be almost, but not quite as black as the Risotto Nero on page 46. Some Portuguese cooks add slices of *chouriço* to the dish too, which is delicious.

Cajun Blackened Catfish

Legendary chef Paul Prudhomme is credited with popularising Cajun cuisine in the US. He is also largely responsible for the famous 'blackened' fish recipes now to be found in restaurants all over the world serving authentic Southern food. Experiment with the quantities for the rub: the final dish should be spicy, so add as much cayenne pepper as you're comfortable with. Don't be tempted to use oil instead of butter, it's the combination of that, and the subsequent dry frying, that gives the cooked fish an appetising blackened appearance.

4 fillets of catfish (150-200g each)

100g melted butter

For the Cajun rub (these are the proportions given to us by a Cajun chef):

1 teaspoon dried thyme

1 teaspoon dried oregano

2 teaspoon onion powder

2 teaspoon garlic powder

1/2 teaspoon cayenne

3 teaspoon sweet paprika

1/2 teaspoon black pepper

1/2 teaspoon salt

1/2 teaspoon ground cumin (optional)

1. Mix all the dry rub ingredients together (cumin wasn't in the original recipe, but we think it works well).

2. Dip the catfish fillets into the melted butter and then coat with the dry rub.

3. Heat a large cast-iron (or other heavy) pan until smoking hot and then add the fillets one by one. If you have a heavy enough pan, you'll probably be able to remove the pan from the heat as soon as the fillets have been added. This is not a bad idea, since you want them to be blackened, not burnt.

4. When nicely blackened on one side, turn over briefly and present, blackened side up.

5. You can serve this with potatoes, if you like, but it's also particularly nice in a sandwich with coleslaw (and is as good cold, if not better, than it is hot).

Horse Mackerel Escabeche

We're big fans of canned sardines. A small can mashed with an equal quantity of unsalted butter, a generous pinch of cayenne and some lemon juice makes a wonderful impromptu fish pâté (or fish paste, depending on your guests). There's a great summary of the history of the sardine canning industry in a piece entitled 'Oules of Sardines' in Elizabeth David's *An Omelette and a Glass of Wine*, where she points out that the process is really just an industrial version of a recipe long practised all over Europe, in which fried fish are preserved under a layer of oil, along the lines of the confit recipe on page 233

This version uses horse mackerel, but you could use sardines, pilchards or any other oily fish. We generally grill our horse mackerel (see below) but this is a nice recipe if you have too much for one meal. Grill the day you buy them, eat the escabeche a week later.

1kg horse mackerel, cleaned

neutral oil for frying

equal quantities of white wine vinegar and water (it's hard to be precise, but you want enough to barely cover the fish once it is placed in a dish or jar for serving)

4 cloves of garlic, finely chopped

1 onion, finely chopped

a pinch of sugar

bay leaf

sprig of parsley

1 red chilli

salt and some whole black peppercorns

extra virgin olive oil for preserving

1. Pan fry the fish in olive or sunflower oil until cooked.

2. Lay the fish in the dish in which you are going to keep them (separate jars is a nice idea).

3. In a separate saucepan add the white wine vinegar, water and all the other ingredients, bring to the boil and cook for 15 to 20 minutes.

4. Pour it hot over the fish and then, when the mixture has cooled, add a layer of extra virgin olive oil so that the fish is kept airtight.

The dish will keep for up to a week (it will probably last longer, but it never gets the chance to in either of our households).

Les Bulots (Whelks)

Let's not beat about the bush here. A helping of highly seasoned, freshly boiled whelks, served just cooled with a bowl of homemade mayonnaise and some French bread, is one of the greatest dishes known to humankind. And even better, the British Isles are, not to put too fine a point on it, Whelk Central. A recent estimate suggests that 10,000 tonnes of whelks are landed in the UK each year. But nearly all of those get exported to South-East Asia. Why? Molluscophobia?

Possibly. But we suspect the same old suspicions and fears that have prompted us to write this book. These are the same suspicions and fears that are partly, at least, responsible for the fact that, in this country, an island, we import £3 million pounds worth of fish each year. That's almost twice the value of fish we imported ten years ago. It makes no sense. The Slow Fish campaign puts it like this:

> With fishing, just as with agriculture, Slow Food strongly believes that every individual can contribute in his or her own small way to changing the mechanisms of a globalised food system based on the intensive exploitation of resources.
>
> Slow Food, with its strong local and international experience, is convinced that we can only bring about change by returning to the origins of food, putting curiosity and pleasure at the service of responsible choices.
>
> We are rediscovering different, forgotten flavours, which the globalised market tends to obliterate, and new or updated recipes. We are seeking to recover the traditional wisdom of fishing communities, who often have not moved far from ancient fishing practices, the diets of past generations, and the known and unknown resources guarded by rivers, lakes and seas. All these things are part of our story and our identity.

Exactly.

A live whelk is a beautiful, beautiful thing; a shelled whelk looks pretty disgusting. You would think, then, that fishmongers would be desperate to make the 5 per cent that remain for the English market as beautifully appetising as possible. Alas, it is nigh on impossible to buy live whelks at fishmongers along the south coast of England (though in the Dieppe fish shops they are all sold live). Instead, they are sold already cooked and shelled (ugly and unappetising); cooked, shelled and pre-frozen (ugly, unappetising and tasteless); or cooked, shelled and heavily pickled in vinegar (ugly, unappetising, tasteless and, ultimately, inedible).

Let's try and get live whelks back on the fish shop counters. Boiled for a couple of minutes and served warm with garlic butter, or cold with mayonnaise, they are delicious. They're also gorgeous tossed in a light dressing made with malt vinegar too, but this is a long way from some of the pickled whelks you find in some 'fresh seafood' stalls. Removed live from the shell, finely sliced and tossed in olive oil, with garlic and lemon, they are simply perfect. In one of his TV shows, Rick Stein stir-fries them with garlic, ginger, spring onion and soy sauce. Whichever way you decide to eat them, let's bring whelks back to the table!

GRILLED FISH

Grilling is one of the most delicious ways of cooking fish. It's also one of the hardest to get right. Most modern cookers are fitted with electric or gas 'grills', but the results you get from placing a fish or fish fillet under one of these grills, and bringing it to the internal temperature required for it to be cooked, are unlikely to resemble properly grilled fish. The problem is that domestic grills never reach the kind of temperature that is required to give you those flecks of char that proper grilling gives, and nor do you get that gentle, charcoal taste. And, to be honest, since domestic cookers are so well adapted to roasting and baking fish we honestly think you'd be better off just using the grill for sausages and bacon (since you can't 'grill' steak under them either).

To us, grilling fish necessarily involves charcoal. Of course, that usually entails cooking outdoors, but it doesn't follow that grilling is a technique only for those in warm climates. Setting up a charcoal grill under cover somewhere is really not so difficult and as long as you keep the grill properly ventilated (carbon monoxide is not nice) there's little that can go wrong.

One more thing about grilled fish is that, with one or two notable exceptions, fish for grilling should always be whole fish. Fish steaks, no matter how much you baste them, have a tendency to dry out when cooked this way. There are some varieties that only come in steaks, it's true, but neither tuna nor swordfish are particularly sustainable (in fact some varieties of both are an absolute no-no). In any case, there are so many smaller, ugly fish available, why bother?

The joy of eating small, whole grilled fish is, sadly, a joy many of us never experience. In Portugal, one of us remembers the sardine season arriving and the joy of the local school children as – at a local event to celebrate – they were each given a salty, grilled sardine on a small bread roll. The children slurped the flesh from the bones, which they then sucked to remove every last morsel. We joked at the time that in the UK such an activity would be frowned upon by the Health and Safety people, but the reality is that many Brits baulk at even the sight of a fish that looks like a fish, let alone the thought of putting one in their mouth and eating it.

We'd like to encourage people to think again, and to question these irrational prejudices. Eat ugly fish. Lick those bones clean!

Tips on grilling fish

It goes without saying that you need a charcoal grill. Don't go out and spend a fortune, just find one that is pretty heavy-duty and reasonably portable. One of the many happy consequences of the recent influx of Eastern European people to the UK, many of whom are experienced grillers of meat and fish, is that many local shops now sell reasonably priced grills aimed precisely at this new market (one of us recently bought a low, home-made Lithuanian 'box' charcoal grill, which is fantastic). The bucket grills found in garden centres and larger supermarkets are also quite good, and handily portable, but we'd encourage you to seek out, or at least look at, the home-made varieties.

As far as preparing the grill goes, most people know that you don't start cooking on a charcoal grill until the embers are glowing white. We find it easier to achieve an even layer of white embers not by delicately arranging the charcoal over the whole of the grill (as some people do) and lighting it, but rather by lumping all the charcoal into a large pile at one end and lighting that. Once the charcoal has burned down, you can then begin moving embers into the cooking area as and when you need them. Keeping the embers on the move is also a good way of regulating the temperature. If it's getting too hot under your fish, simply move the embers away.

Aside from that it's always a good idea to have at least two height positions, one close(ish) to the embers, one higher (but this is easily improvised with a few stones or pebbles). You will also need a small assortment of those folding wire fish baskets. The ones with wooden handles are nice, but since wood doesn't understand the crucial difference between grilling and being grilled, we suggest all metal. When grilling fish, use these all the time. If you do, you will never, ever need to try and turn a fish on the bars of a grill again.

As for plates, knives, forks and so on, you won't need any because you're going to eat with your fingers. If you feel you simply have to have something on which to present your cooked fish, find a large flat pebble or a piece of driftwood. Hugh Fearnley-Whittingstall suggests sending the kids off to find smooth pebble 'plates' and we think that's a fine idea. Washing your hands in the sea is fun too.

Small fish are much easier to grill than large ones and 500g is probably a sensible upper limit, but many of the fish we list below will never reach that size. The best fish for grilling are those with a relatively high fat content, and this rules out pollack, whiting and the like. Strangely, we had success with

Dover sole and chargrilled turbot is also a dish of rare beauty (quite odd really, because baked in the oven turbot has a tendency to dry out). We find that adding a generous sprinkling of sea-salt to our fish before we cook it not only adds a salty tang – recall, we do like our food properly seasoned – but also firms up the flesh a little. Some of our favourites are:

Black bream

Grilled black bream is a revelation. Seriously, it's up there with sea bass, gilt-head bream and all those other marine heavyweights. Try it. You will not be disappointed.

Horse mackerel

This is almost universally despised in the UK (where it is also known as scad), but highly prized in Portugal, where it is known as *carapau*. It's also very popular in Japan, and they really know their fish. Salt it generously before you grill it. It's bony, yes, but fish are. Get over it.

Garfish

> All tail and proboscis... this miserable sea-worm with verdigris-tinted spine...
>
> Douglas, N. *Siren Land*, 1911

Garfish tastes remarkably like mackerel. In fact, they often swim with mackerel shoals. Once you have devoured the flesh do not be disturbed by the fact that the bones are a rather conspicuous greenish-blue. The true eel-pout (don't get us started on that again) also has green-blue bones. Chemists in Germany recently ascribed the colour to the presence of biliverdin, the bile pigment also responsible for the greenish colour sometimes found in bruises.

Stone bass (wreckfish)

This is one of the exceptions to the recommendation we mention above. Stone bass grow to up to two metres in length, so it's unlikely you'll ever grill one whole. Cut into thick steaks, however, they are perfect for the grill. The oil content of the flesh is similar to that of sea bass, a fish to which it is related, and we suppose it is this that prevents it drying out. It is very popular in Portugal, where it is known as *cherne*. Pour extra virgin olive oil over the cooked fish and garnish with thin slices of raw garlic.

Sardine

Sardines are not ugly at all. In fact, they (like herrings) are absolutely beautiful. We mention them here because, in many ways, they are the perfect grilling fish. We eat them as the Portuguese do. Place one grilled sardine in a bread roll roughly the same length as the fish and eat: head, tail, bones and all.

Rabbit

Rabbits aren't ugly either, and, well, they're not fish (although the Medieval Catholic church did consider them honorary fish for the purposes of Friday abstinence, along with beavers and capybara, but that's a story for another chapter). Since rabbit responds well to slow char-grilling in a way that no other meats in this volume do, we thought we'd mention it here. Marinate the legs and saddles in olive oil, lemon juice and salt for a couple of hours. Grill slowly over white coals and, when it's nearly cooked, thread liver, heart and kidneys onto wooden skewers and grill briefly (and don't forget to pre-soak the skewers in water so they don't char).

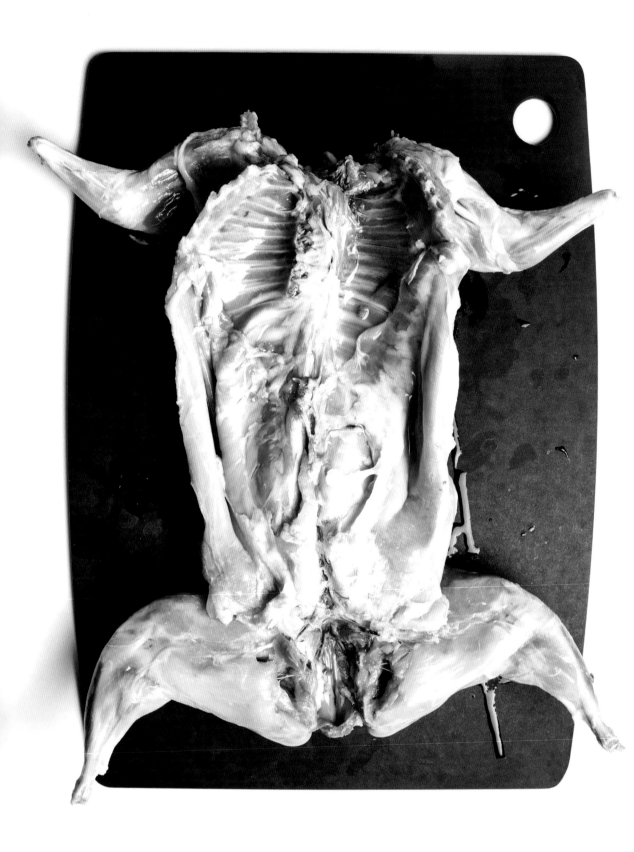

5. RABBITS AND SQUIRRELS

A tail of two cuties

If you are looking for overlooked, sustainable ingredients, you can't do much better than rabbits and (grey) squirrels. These little critters breed prodigiously, and in many countries their numbers have reached (or at least once reached) problem proportions. In October 1859, Thomas Austin – a landowner and farmer in Victoria, Australia – introduced twenty-four breeding rabbits into the local habitat, mostly to satisfy his penchant for shooting parties. Eighteen months later, he wrote in a letter to The Acclimatisation Society:

> I have done a little myself towards introducing game birds. I brought out in the Yorkshire nine hares and thirty-four black-birds and thrushes, which I am going to turn out here, and my man, this last season, has reared about seventy pheasants: some have bred out in their natural way; and I have seen two coveys of partridges, one of six young ones, the other eight; and the English wild rabbit I have in thousands...

And yet, by 1870, around 2 million rabbits were being killed or shot every year in Australia without making even a dent in the population. Every year at Easter, the South Island of New Zealand hosts a bunny-shooting bonanza as part of its pest control measures. In 2016, the cull netted 10,000 rabbits over 24 hours; the record is more than twice that. Sadly, it was reported that most of the rabbits were used as fertiliser, and some taken home to feed pets. Only 'a few keen foodies' claimed any for the pot. What a waste.

With their prodigious breeding rate, it's perhaps no wonder that Pope Francis, when searching for a suitable comparison, told Catholics recently that they should avoid breeding 'like rabbits'. His comments caused some offence – to rabbit breeders. The president of the German Rabbit Breeders

Association told the media that the Pope should allow Catholics to use contraception rather than resorting to misleading clichés about rabbits.

Rabbits can be hunted in the wild, but they can also be bred in captivity. There are a number of factors that make rabbit rearing an attractive proposition. The breeding rate is an obvious one, but there are others: firstly, the meat is incredibly healthy – a rabbit carcass contains only 7 per cent fat, compared with figures of over 30 per cent for pigs, sheep and cattle; secondly, rabbits turn 20 per cent of the feed they consume into edible meat, compared to 18 per cent for pigs and 16 per cent for cattle; thirdly, they take up very little space, are very easily looked after and easily transportable should the plan be to sell them; finally (a point often overlooked), they thrive on cellulose-rich plants, such as grass, which means they are not in direct competition with humans for food – domestic poultry, for example, eat grain. The Food and Agriculture Organization of the United Nations (FAO) have proposed that this final factor is one of the reasons small-scale 'backyard rabbitries' may be part of the answer to projected global food shortages (*The Rabbit: Husbandry, Health and Production*, 1997). Be aware, though, that these factors have also made intensive rabbit breeding an attractive proposition, and that some rabbits are reared in very poor conditions; more on this below.

We want to do our bit to get wild and humanely-farmed rabbit eaten more regularly. Rabbit tastes great and is really easy to prepare and cook. It's not surprising that it remains very popular in much of Europe. The Greeks make a sensational slow-cooked *stifado* from rabbits and onions (recipe on page 163); the French have all manner of delicious rabbit recipes; subtly-spiced, slow-braised rabbit often forms the scented centrepiece to a Moroccan feast. And as well as this, you can use virtually the whole beast, including the ears (what could be called 'nose to cottontail eating'). Deep fried rabbit ears with aromatic herbs, which was a classic snack at the world-acclaimed Catalan restaurant El Bulli, is a cinch to do at home, and utterly delicious (recipe, p. 178). Spicy rabbit heads are a succulent Sichuanese delicacy.

So why are rabbits rarely eaten in Anglo-Saxon cuisines, and squirrels not at all? Well, actually, they once were: rabbit casserole used to be widely cooked and eaten in the UK; the meat content of that speciality of the south east of the US – Brunswick stew – was originally rabbit or squirrel, but nowadays most people prepare it with chicken. In his hugely entertaining book *The Tenth Muse* (1954) Sir Harry Luke reports that at picnics in the southern states of the US the guest of honour was typically served with the brain of a barbecued squirrel.

As food production has become more industrial, and game meats have gone from being a treat to something to be suspicious of, rabbit is no longer a regular part of most people's diets. The spread of myxomatosis in the 1950s doubtless didn't help. This deadly viral disease gives rabbits skin tumours and blindness and decimated their populations until immunity developed and numbers began to rebound. (Note that myxomatosis is harmless to humans, and does not affect the safety of rabbit meat.)

In this chapter we dig into the mythology and facts surrounding rabbits and squirrels. Did you know, for example, that understanding the breeding patterns of rabbits can provide deep and mysterious insight into the structures of leaves and lungs, how to most effectively organise your warehouse, and the secrets of good photographic composition? We reveal how a twelfth-century rabbit-fancier discovered one of the most powerful of mathematical insights while trying to work out his bunny production rate. We also reveal how rabbit milk could be a medicinal marvel, and the strange properties of rabbit urine.

We want you to take another look at rabbits, and grey squirrels too. They are fascinating animals, and a tasty, cheap and sustainable alternative to mass produced meats.

One important note of caution, though. In some places in Europe, the remarkable breeding rates of rabbits have been exploited in order to mass produce them – sometimes in very poor conditions. By far the largest producers of farmed rabbits in the European Union are Italy, Spain and France and much of the rabbit sold in the UK is imported – nearly all of this farmed. While some producers raise rabbits in less intensive pens, many use extremely small barren cages. This is bad for animal welfare, and bad for the quality of the meat. There is currently no EU legislation specifically regulating the welfare of farmed rabbits. When buying rabbit, it is therefore important to know the source; see the Raising and Butchering Basics section for more.

Rodent redux

James Gidley was sceptical. The prominent American palaeontologist was sitting at his desk at the National Museum of Natural History, looking at teeth – fossil teeth – and thinking about rabbits. Their dental structure (and that of their hare cousins) was clearly different from all other rodents. And after much searching of the fossil record, and examination of modern-day skeletons of different species, he could find no other features that showed they evolved from a common rodent ancestor. Ever since Linnaeus, rabbits had been classified together with rodents in the order Rodentia. In fact, almost any mammal with long front teeth had been uncritically added to this order, but in the case of rabbits and hares and pikas, he was sure this was wrong. He penned a short, two-page article for the journal *Science*, published in 1912, setting out the case for separating these animals into a separate order Lagomorpha. His arguments were widely accepted, and led to many other academics proposing that other rodents should be reclassified, and to claims that lagomorphs and rodents weren't even closely related (modern genetic techniques have established that they are, and that rodents do form a single grouping).

Rodents aren't just prolific, they're everywhere: almost half of all species of mammals are rodents. So it's hardly surprising that they form a staple part of many people's diets. The Romans cherished dormice, and some Italians do today. Venezuelans are partial to capybara – the largest rodent in the world. Peruvians and Bolivians love guinea pigs, and they are so entrenched in food culture that a famous painting of the Last Supper in Cusco Cathedral in the Andes depicts Christ and his disciples dining on guinea pig. But in British cuisine, rodents are generally rejected, and even their close relation the rabbit is regarded with suspicion by most consumers – a speciality game item for the adventurous, but not an everyday meal. We are surrounded by rabbits and squirrels, but we don't eat them. This has nothing to do with how these creatures taste, and everything to do with appearances and culturally-determined reputations.

One oft-cited reason is that they are too cute to eat, particularly fluffy bunnies. When the author of the respected food blog *Hungry in Hogtown* posted an article on cooking rabbit ears (recipe on page 178), the reaction was intense – with commenters hoping that the author 'died from rabbit syphilis' (medically impossible, as it happens) or 'choked to death' or asking 'how can you sleep at night?' The author wrote a follow-up post to explain that eating all parts of the animal was a mark of respect, reduced needless waste, and that the animal-welfare aspects of eating rabbit were likely much less than eating chicken or non-free-range eggs. We suspect that the idea of eating squirrels will engender a similarly shocked reaction in many people.

But why? As we say in the introduction, we think all this fussiness has little to do with aesthetics, and much more to do with Western society's increasingly unhealthy cultural relationship with food. Meat and fish is now viewed as a processed product, like chocolate or cheese. It should come shrink-wrapped, ready to use, with as little blood as possible, and definitely no cheeks or feet. And just as processed cheese and mass produced chocolate are insipid, so it is with meat. It should, preferably, taste as little as possible of flesh: commercial supermarket chicken breast is a brine-saturated mass of tasteless texture, and the least piggy-tasting parts of the pig – the fillet and chops – are the preferred cuts. As if this were not enough, these tasteless products must also be cooked into submission. A chicken breast is tender and juicy when cooked to an internal temperature of 60°C, but most people are used to the dry, less-flavourful results of chicken cooked to a much higher temperature – 75°C or 80°C. The same is true of pork. The US Food Safety and Inspection Service recommends a minimum temperature of 74°C for chicken breast – not so much for food safety reasons, apparently, as to conform to consumer preference (see Nathan Myhrvold, Chris Young and Maxime Bilet, 'Yes, you are overcooking your food', *Scientific American*, 2011).

All in all, it seems that the consumer has become squeamish about animal and fish products: the less the food we buy looks like animal or fish, the better; and the milder the taste, the better. This is wasteful, and it encourages unhealthy and unsustainable food production methods. It also means that unusual food sources – particularly creatures that prompt an emotional reaction, positive or negative – are shunned. Like rabbit and squirrel.

It was not always so. One of us remembers a sign outside a rural butcher's shop in the late-70s declaring 'Watership Down: You've seen the movie, now eat the pie'. Consumers were amused, and sales of rabbit pie were brisk. By the early-90s, things had changed. When *Spy Magazine* in the US decided to construct an elaborate hoax (April 1992 edition) to show that PR firms would take on any campaign, however impossible, as long as the price was right, the doomed product that they concocted was the bunny burger! (We provide a fabulous recipe on page 176) The magazine, posing as Bunny Burgers Inc., asked for help 'mitigating public hostility toward the consumption of bunny meat at a time of burgeoning sensitivity toward the animals with whom we share this fragile planet', fearing that 'PR firms would hang up on us when we phoned to describe our fictitious enterprise'. None did. *Spy Magazine* was shocked. Passers-by in a New Jersey mall who were subsequently invited to try a bunny burger reacted mostly with alarm and revulsion: 'Rabbits are cute little things', said one, 'Not like cows'. Actually, the burgers being handed out were made of turkey – even *Spy Magazine* wouldn't go so far, it seems, as to offer unsuspecting members of the public a burger made of real rabbit.

It's the same with squirrel. When a north London branch of Budgens supermarket started selling grey squirrel a few years ago, it found that some customers were intrigued by what was billed as a 'tasty and sustainable' alternative meat. They sold a couple of squirrels per day, but also came in for some flak, with the animal welfare group Viva accusing the store of 'having the blood of a beautiful wild animal on their hands' and of 'profiting from a wildlife massacre'. Why, then, no concern about the large quantities of farmed meat on sale at the store, also from beautiful animals?

Squirrel squeamishness

Squirrels, perhaps because of their ubiquity, seem generally to have been taken for granted. In folk culture, they are often portrayed as mischievous or thieving. In Norse mythology, the squirrel Ratatosk is a gossipy creature that flits up and down the world tree Yggdrasil, making trouble between the eagle at the top and the serpent at the bottom. Ratatosk also spied for Odin. Perhaps it is this suspicion about squirrel espionage that has fuelled the rise of anti-squirrel extremist groups in the US such as North American Defence against Squirrels (NADS) and the Anti-Squirrel Coalition.

In the indigenous Japanese Ainu culture, squirrel meat was thought to have special powers to help those needing new teeth (hardly a huge leap of the imagination) and as a cure for infertility (perhaps slightly less obvious). The Kwakiutl tribe of British Colombia fed small pieces of squirrel heart to infant males to imbue them with the ability as hunters to dash with lightning speed from one place to another. Squirrel fat was also reputed to be a cure for earache and toothache (if you want to give this a go, you might want to try the rillettes recipe on page 160). These and many other interesting facts can be found in Kim Long's *Squirrels: A Wildlife Handbook*.

Squirrels have been an important source of food in tough times, as they don't hibernate and therefore provide a year-round protein supply. They can also do damage to crops and so were often killed by farming communities, therefore ending up in the pot. But they are no longer regularly eaten in most places.

Like rabbits, squirrels are cute too. But in the UK, there is a hefty dose of racial discrimination involved: the native red squirrels are seen as attractive, charming and meek; the immigrant grey squirrels have been portrayed as aggressive interlopers. Indeed, English law prohibits anyone who captures a grey squirrel from releasing it, in order to preserve the native reds. With a grey squirrel population of more than 2 million, outnumbering reds by some 20 to 1, one can't help but feel this is the kind of populist legislation typical of immigration issues. But what is clear is that a lot of good, sustainable meat is going to waste. If you are required to kill the grey squirrel that has become trapped in your bird-feeder, at least have the decency to confit it afterwards (recipe on page 158).

This was an approach explicitly advocated for in the UK's House of Lords. Now, it must be recalled that the upper house is comprised mostly of unelected Peers, a number of whom have inherited their titles from days of yore, and that many of them own vast tracts of the British countryside. They wear ceremonial gowns made traditionally from short-tailed weasel (known euphemistically as 'ermine', to rhyme with 'vermin'); but nowadays mostly made from the weasel's favourite prey, the rabbit.

So perhaps it shouldn't be all that surprising that in 2006, the Lords devoted more than 2.5 hours of their parliamentary time to a debate on squirrels. Although ridiculed in advance in the British press, member after member stood up to congratulate the Lord who initiated the debate, praising his 'courage' and affirming the importance of the issue. A full account can be found in the *Hansard* (23 March 2006, column 355 onwards to be precise).

At stake was the very fate of the beloved native red squirrel, under existential threat from an 'American invader', the grey squirrel. The house had to weigh several different policy options. Aware that many people regarded the grey squirrel as being cute, much time was devoted to vilification: Lord Redesdale stated that they were 'rats with good PR'; Lord Hoyle confirmed that one had recently 'run up my leg and bit me'; Lady Saltoun of Abernethy noted that 'red squirrels are rather like quiet, well behaved people, who do not make a nuisance or an exhibition of themselves, or commit crimes, and so do not get themselves into the papers in the vulgar way grey squirrels do'; and Lord Monro of Langholm pointed out that they were a nuisance to car-owners: 'they stand on the roof and do all sorts of things on the windscreen'.

There was a sense of shared outrage. But what to do? Lady Saltoun raised the possibility of eating them, and hit the nail on the head when she worried that even if edible, 'it would be rather difficult to establish the market because a lot of people, children in particular, would say, "Oh no, I couldn't possibly eat that", just as they say they cannot eat dear little bunny rabbits'. Lord Inglewood confirmed that they were indeed edible, recalling the adventures of Sir Stephen Tallents, who saw a grey squirrel in his garden one day.

> The squirrel was shot ... As I skinned it, I seemed to remember that in America squirrel, fried or stewed was a favoured dish. So next morning I rang up the Natural History Museum to inquire if I could safely eat my grey squirrel's remains. The Museum was courteous but diffident, and promised to ring up the Zoo. The Zoo, I learned, was encouraging but could not speak from first-hand knowledge. I wavered, but a man on my homeward train told me of a lady who in those wartime days was feeding boiled grey squirrel to her dogs. That was good enough to me.

Taking this as his cue, the noble Lord suggested putting squirrels on school menus, or even on the menu of the Peers' Dining Room, noting that there was a precedent (his father, shortly after the War, had found 'black partridge' on the parliamentary menu, 'which had turned out after some investigation to be young rook'). But he realised that this would not be enough given the scale of the problem, and therefore extended an invitation to all the relevant members of government:

> ...to the hotel in the Lake District where I am a director – and which has, I hasten to add, one AA rosette for fine food – to dine on grey squirrels to launch an "Eat a grey to save a red" campaign. I will feel very let down and be very sceptical of the Government's true intentions on biodiversity if, on the advice of some politically correct adviser, the invitation is refused. After all, let us not forget that many of the things we eat as a matter of course are entirely lovable and pretty creatures which appeal to the wider world.

We couldn't have put it better ourselves.

Nut and Bolts: the truth about rabbits and squirrels

Rabbits and squirrels are amazing creatures. Here are some bizarre facts to bedazzle your dinner party guests with while they're waiting for the dinner to slow cook:

1. *Despite their long front teeth, rabbits are not rodents.* Squirrels are. Well, ok, you probably did know that because we talked about it in the last section.

2. *Squirrels sometimes turn carnivorous. Rabbits don't.* While squirrels mainly eat a vegetarian diet, some will also consume meat, especially when hungry. They have been known to eat insects, eggs, small birds and smaller rodents. The cute squirrel has even been known to engage in cannibalism. Rabbits, however, are herbivores. Except for that killer bunny in Monty Python and the Holy Grail.

3. *Squirrels like rattlesnake gore.* It's true. California ground squirrels love nothing better than finding a dead rattlesnake or shed skin, giving it a good chomp, and then licking themselves all over. While it may sound fetishist, there is actually a good explanation. These squirrels live in burrows rather than trees, putting them at particular risk of predation by snakes. Their ingenious response is to mask their own smell with snake scent, particularly useful when they are asleep in their burrows. Predatory snakes are tricked into believing that the burrow is full of rattlesnake rather than a fluffy meal.

4. *Rabbits have testicles in front of their penis. Squirrels don't.* Feel free to confirm this next time you're at the pet shop; but maybe you should just trust us on this one. There's another thing you should trust us on –

rather than, say, Googling it at work – which is that male Cape ground squirrels have massive testicles and extremely long penises. Around 40 per cent of their body length, to be precise (we'll let you do the maths to work out how that compares). They put this to good medical use by auto-fellating themselves after intercourse, probably as a way of flushing out the genital tract to prevent sexually-transmitted infections, according to scientists.

5. *Squirrels build nests in trees. Rabbits don't.* These nests, made by tree squirrels and flying squirrels, are known as 'dreys'. They can be a foot or more in diameter, made of twigs and lined with softer materials. Squirrels either spend a huge amount of time building and maintaining a drey, or sometimes steal someone else's.

6. *Squirrel brain bonjela.* An old remedy for teething babies was to rub their gums with squirrel brains. Brains have no known analgesic properties, but if someone smashed open a squirrel's head and shoved the goo in your mouth, you'd probably shut up too.

7. *Rabbits are a kind of fish.* Well, to be clear, scientists definitely do not regard rabbits as a kind of fish. But the Medieval Catholic church did – it wasn't, after all, an institution known for being concerned about doctrine conflicting with science. Posterity records that in 600 AD Pope Gregory I authorised the consumption of laurices (foetal or baby rabbits) during Lent and other fast days, declaring them to be – all evidence to the contrary notwithstanding – a marine species like fish and shellfish. This was no doubt a great relief to the monastic orders, who at the time had to observe more than 180 fast days per year, and who were keen cuniculturists (breeders of rabbits). The edict was later annulled, but under pressure from their flocks in the Americas, subsequent popes saw fit to authorise the consumption of beavers and capybara on fast days, on the basis that they lived some of their lives in water...

8. *Toothy terrors.* Squirrel incisors grow about 6 inches (15 cm) per year. The only thing that stops them turning into Scary Sabretooth Squirrels is that the teeth are worn away by continual gnawing. Scary Sabretooth Squirrels did actually once exist, though. Their scientific name is Cronopio dentiacutus and they lived 60 million years ago. And they did look pretty scary (a Google image search will confirm).

9. *Rabbit show-jumping is a popular sport in many countries.* It is particularly big in Sweden, where it originated and is called *kaninhopning*.

It became so popular that a Swedish Federation of Rabbit Jumping was established as the sport's governing body. It sets rules based on horse show jumping but 'adapted to better suit rabbits' – including 'no beating or kicking the rabbit'. Helpful hints on training your rabbit include to put it in front of a jump 'and give it some time to think'.

10. Squirrels have twice been responsible for bringing down the NASDAQ stock market. They did this by chewing through power cables resulting in short circuits that shut down vital electrical equipment.

Medicinal marvel?

Rabbit cheese is reputed to have medicinal qualities. And no, we haven't been watching Monty Python. According to Pliny, the Roman natural philosopher, rabbit milk makes a superlative cheese that can cure diarrhoea.

> Cheese cannot be made from the milk of animals which have teeth on either jaw, from the circumstance that their milk does not coagulate. … The rennet of the fawn, the hare, and the kid is the most esteemed, but the best of all is that of the dasypus [rabbit]: this last acts as a specific for diarrhoea, that animal being the only one with teeth in both jaws, the rennet of which has that property.

Pliny's *Natural History*, Book XI, Chapter 97

We have no idea how to milk a rabbit. But Dutch farmers do, because 2000 years after Pliny penned his thoughts on cheese, medicinal rabbit milk is making a comeback. The Dutch biotech company Pharming has genetically engineered rabbits to produce in their milk a therapeutic protein that can treat angioedema – a condition causing episodes of severe and potentially fatal swelling. These rabbits are now being farmed at a commercial scale. Each rabbit produces about 120 ml of milk per day, obtained through mini pumping machines. According to *National Geographic*, it's just like a dairy farm 'but on a smaller scale'. US company LBF is using rabbits that produce the essential blood clotting agent Factor VII to treat haemophilia.

Rabbits and the Meaning of Life

But enough about bodily excretions. Let's talk about sex. It turns out that understanding the breeding patterns of rabbits can provide deep and mysterious insight into the structures of leaves and lungs and how to most effectively organise your warehouse. When the medieval merchant and mathematician Fibonacci sat down to calculate bunny production rates, his solution to the problem became one of the most famous discoveries in mathematics.

Here was the problem he laid out in his 1202 book *Liber abaci* ('book of calculation'):

> A pair of newborn rabbits, male and female, are put in a field. Rabbits are able to mate at the age of one month and have a gestation period of one month, so that at the end of the second month, the female will give birth. Suppose that each female produces one new pair (a male and a female) every month from the age of two months and that all rabbits survive the first year. How many pairs will there be after one year?

As Fibonacci showed, the number of pairs of rabbits each month is given by the following sequence, where each number is the sum of the two that precede it:

1, 1, 2, 3, 5, 8, 13, 21, 34, 55, 89, 144, 233

So there are 233 pairs of rabbits after a year (the thirteenth number in the sequence – since the first number is the population at the beginning, the second number after one month, and the thirteenth number after twelve months). That's quite a lot of confit, but also quite a lot of inbreeding – so do try to swap bunnies with your friends. It's also a conservative estimate, as the average litter size for rabbits is around six (although not every female will breed every month).

So Thomas Austin wasn't exaggerating when eighteen months after introducing (adult) rabbits to Australia he claimed to have 'thousands'. The eighteenth number in the Fibonacci sequence is 2584, and since he started with twelve pairs we should probably take the twenty-fifth number (7 + 18, since the seventh number is closest to twelve) which is a staggering 75,025.

This sequence of Fibonacci numbers (which was known to the Indian mathematicians of antiquity) crops up in all sorts of natural phenomena – the number of petals on some flowers is always a Fibonacci number (so daisies can have 13, 21, 34, 55 or 89 petals). The interlocked spirals of seeds that make up sunflower heads also follow the Fibonacci sequence, with the number of spirals to the left and the number to the right almost always being adjacent Fibonacci numbers. The same is true of pine cone and pineapple scales. Trees and plants grow in a binary branching manner, and the number of leaves or branches at each stage (assuming none drop off or fail to develop) is a Fibonacci number.

It turns out that making use of the Fibonacci sequence is the most efficient way to pack a space (with seeds, petals, leaves or pineapple scales) and keep filling that space as the size grows. This is why evolution has led many organisms to settle on it – and why modern warehouses make use of it. Cauliflower heads and lungs follow the same principle in three dimensions. But one shouldn't get carried away. Some flowers have other numbers of petals, and the oft-repeated claim that the spiral of snail shells and sea shells is perfectly described by the Fibonacci sequence looks plausible in computer simulations, but falls flat if one measures actual shells.

But now we are becoming distracted from our rabbits, and should cook some before they start breeding.

Buying rabbit and squirrel

Squirrel remains a speciality game meat that can be hard to find in butchers and supermarkets. We hope that this book can help to change that, but in the meantime, it is available from some game butchers, or you can order it online from our friends at The Wild Meat Company (wildmeat.co.uk) – who also have a fantastic range of other products, including wild rabbit. Squirrel is not seasonal game, and can be found all year round. Young squirrels are the most tender; older specimens require longer cooking.

Rabbit meat is not too difficult to find in the UK, but be aware that much if it is imported from the Continent or from China – and most imported rabbit is cage-reared. Ask your butcher where the rabbit comes from and how the animal was raised, or check supermarket labelling carefully. (As far as we are aware, no one – yet – is farming squirrels.)

Some people have concerns about wild rabbits having myxomatosis. There is nothing to worry about. The virus only affects rabbits, and does not lead to any food safety issues. Food safety inspections also mean that a diseased rabbit is very unlikely to enter the supply chain in any case.

Buy wild rabbit if you possibly can. Unlike some other game, there is no closed season for rabbit and it is available all year round. Wild rabbits tend to be smaller and leaner, and can be a little tougher (especially older ones), but you will have no difficulty achieving tender, succulent results if you follow our cooking tips – and the taste of wild rabbit is incomparable. However, in some areas demand outstrips supply – not helped by the fact that much wild UK rabbit meat is sold for export. If you are having difficulty finding it locally, order online from The Wild Meat Company (there are a few other game butchers who will also do mail-order deliveries).

If you do buy farmed rabbit, we strongly recommend buying meat that is certified organic, or (if you can find it) free-range. Failing this, buy the meat of rabbits that have been reared in pens, not cages. If rabbit meat is not specifically labelled as wild (game) rabbit or as organic, free-range or reared in pens, then it is very likely to have been produced in battery cages and we advise that you do not buy it. But you always have the option of rearing or catching your own rabbits.

Raising and butchering basics

Here is everything you need to know about procuring, preparing and cooking rabbits and squirrels yourself.

Welfare concerns for farmed rabbits

While rabbit is still something of a speciality meat in the UK, it is much more widely eaten on the Continent. In fact, some 326 million rabbits are farmed for their meat in Europe every year – mostly in Italy, Spain and France. This has led some producers to adopt highly intensive farming techniques. Unlike most other farmed animals, there is currently no EU legislation specifically regulating the welfare of farmed rabbits.

A recent exposé by the organisation Compassion in World Farming has shed some rather disturbing light on this. Rabbits are regularly kept in tiny, barren battery cages – something that the European Union has banned for hens. This in turn requires massive antibiotic use to control infections. Apart from the disturbing welfare issues involved, the indiscriminate use of antibiotics in farming is a significant contributor to antibiotic resistance, making it a major global public health issue. And naturally, the quality of meat produced in such conditions, with animals that can barely move being reared on a diet of commercial feed and antibiotics, suffers greatly.

There are alternatives, of course, to battery cages. Some producers keep rabbits in straw-lined pens rather than cages, which gives them more space, allows social interactions, and tends to provide more enrichment. Organic production systems rear rabbits in pens with additional access to an area of pasture.

We urge you not to buy cage-reared rabbits. If no information is available on how the animal was raised, it is very likely to be battery farmed, and you should find another source.

Catching

There are plenty of tasty wild rabbits and squirrels scampering around the British countryside – and, most likely, in your back garden. If you have the opportunity and the inclination, why not catch some?

Rabbits and grey squirrels are regarded as pests, and they may be hunted throughout the year – there is no closed season (except on 'moorland and unenclosed land'). All you need is some land or permission to hunt on someone else's land. Squirrels are at their plumpest and tastiest from late summer to early winter. Rabbits are good all year round, but best in the autumn and throughout the winter. Younger, smaller rabbits are generally more tender, but with low, slow cooking used in most of the recipes in this chapter, even older larger rabbits will emerge from the pot tasty and tender.

There are a number of options for catching rabbits and squirrels. For rabbits, hunting with a shotgun is probably the easiest and most humane, provided you have a firearms certificate issued by the police, and the necessary shooting skills. You can shoot in the daytime, or – with certain restrictions – at night-time with lights. It is not practical to use a shotgun in built-up areas and there are certain restrictions on using them within fifty metres of a road (basically, if you endanger someone by doing so, you're in trouble). Bottom line: it's only feasible to hunt with a shotgun in rural areas.

The other option is to use a less-powerful air rifle, which does not require a licence. Provided you do not cause a disturbance and use it responsibly (not firing pellets beyond the boundary of your land, for example), you can shoot rabbits or squirrels with an air rifle in any decent-sized garden. You should get a powerful air rifle, pressurised to the maximum legal limit (12ft lb or 16.25J). Make sure you have the skill to hit your target with a clean shot (a shot to the head is the best, for both humane and culinary reasons) and ensure that you know what the maximum effective range of your gun is. You should also probably have a chat with your neighbours first, and maybe invite them over for rabbit stew occasionally.

It is also possible to use humane cage traps for rabbits or squirrels, with appropriately appetising bait such as carrots or nuts. These should be checked at regular intervals – at least twice a day – to avoid unnecessary suffering and in case a protected species (such as a red squirrel) is inadvertently trapped, so that it can be released unharmed. You should dispatch trapped rabbits and squirrels quickly and humanely (see below) – it is an offence to kill them using a non-humane method. When removing them from a trap, a hessian sack and a good pair of gloves can be invaluable.

If you do trap squirrels, don't get any pangs of remorse and release them – it is actually an offence to keep or release grey squirrels; you are required to kill them humanely if you catch them alive. Eating is optional, but we very much encourage it. Note that red squirrels are a protected species, and it is an offence to kill them.

You can also use ferrets and falcons to catch rabbits. We've never tried either.

One thing to note about squirrels: while rabbits are herbivorous, and wild ones in your garden are very unlikely to have eaten anything other than grass, your herbaceous border, and your vegetable patch, squirrels are semi-omnivorous. In a rural setting with plenty of food choice, squirrels will usually eat mainly nuts and berries – this is one of the reasons they taste so good – perhaps together with the odd opportunistic bird's egg. But in urban environments, they are not averse to rifling through your bins and eating all kinds of scraps and rubbish. This generally isn't dangerous – unless they've eaten someone's rat poison – but we do recommend country squirrel over the inner-city variety.

Raising your own

Rabbits are really very easy to raise yourself. You only need a small amount of space for a pen that they can run around in, a small investment, and the time to care for them properly. Unlike other backyard animals, rabbits make almost no noise, eat a wide variety of food (vegetable scraps, grass, dandelions...) and usually require no specialist veterinary care. They breed well and thrive in the temperate climate of the UK. They are simple to butcher, and much quicker and easier to skin than a bird is to pluck.

There are plenty of websites that can give advice on setting up and maintaining a rabbitry (including the excellent PocketFarm.co.uk and RudolphsRabbitRanch.com). You will need a male (buck) and a couple of females (does), of a suitable breed for eating, such as New Zealand White. You'll ideally need hutches or covered cages with outside runs to provide both protection from the weather and a free-range area. Domesticated breeds have generally lost the urge to dig, so you shouldn't have too many issues with escapes. Fine-mesh wire cages are another possibility, with added weather protection and preferably also with access to an outside run. Indoor cages, large and high enough for the animals to run and jump around in, are also possible, but not ideal for the welfare of the animals. Whichever system you use, you'll need three separated areas: one breeding area, where the buck is kept and where does are brought for mating; one area for each breeding doe and their litter; and another area to move the weaned offspring into until they are big enough to eat.

Commercial pellets are available that provide a balanced and nutritious diet. But if you don't mind your rabbits growing a little more slowly, it's also perfectly possible to feed them on a mixture of grass cuttings, vegetable scraps, foraged greens and so on. They will then reach eating size in three months, instead of two on pellets. Some people use rabbits to mow their lawn, by putting them in portable mesh cages, with a covered area at the end for protection, and moving them around to different areas when they've eaten the grass under their cage. Rabbits should always have a plentiful supply of water available, and a net of hay which aids digestion.

Be careful that you don't get overrun with rabbits. It can happen very easily, given that a doe can produce a litter of six every six weeks, gestation is a month, and the young are weaned at eight weeks. We recommend breeding from your does no more than once every three months. You may also need to separate male and female offspring before they start breeding among themselves, at about 5 to 8 weeks.

In addition to providing a ready supply of delicious meat, keeping rabbits can also be a boon for your garden. As long as you keep them away from your prize vegetables, rabbit droppings make great fertiliser, and their urine is apparently particularly good for citrus trees that need both nitrogen and a low pH.

Squirrels are much trickier to breed than rabbits, because they climb and require a larger cage. They also reputedly have difficulty distinguishing food from the fingers that feed them. Solutions to these and other logistical challenges were worked out by 1910, when the Children's Encyclopaedia explained How to Keep a Pet Squirrel (popularised in an illustrated book by Axel Scheffler published a hundred years later). Unfortunately – or perhaps fortunately – it is illegal to keep wild squirrels without a licence in the UK, and we're not sure you'd get a licence for breeding purposes, since grey squirrels are classed as a pest species. All in all, it's probably not a good idea to set up a squirrel farm.

KILLING AND ITS ETHICAL CONSIDERATIONS

If you are going to set up a rabbitry, you need to be comfortable with the idea of killing rabbits yourself. It is unlikely that anyone will volunteer to come and do it for you.

You might also need to be prepared for some negative reactions to raising rabbits for meat. A quick look at the comments section of online articles on eating rabbit reveals some very strong views. We find this a little odd. Anyone who is uncomfortable with the idea that the food on their plate was once an animal, and that the animal was killed in order for them to eat it, really ought to reconsider whether they should be eating meat at all. But we suspect that many of those expressing shock and horror at the idea of eating bunnies or squirrels are quite happy to tuck into a burger or fast-food fried chicken. It may be uncomfortable to be confronted with the reality that meat comes from a living, breathing animal; but being faced with that reality makes it much harder to take the meat for granted. The worst excesses of the global meat industry take place precisely when we have lost the connection between the living animal and the butchered meat. Meat consumption in certain parts of the Western world now increasingly depends on such a unhealthy disconnect. That vacuum-packed, hormone-saturated skinless chicken breast, or that brine-injected pork tenderloin, could just as easily have been made in a laboratory as removed from an animal's carcass. We find it genuinely odd when our friends tell us how repulsed they are when the see lambs' heads on display in a Greek market: just what do they think is in their shepherd's pie? And as we saw in the introduction, the standards by which people make their food choices are often double standards. Many of the people who are squeamish at the sight of an animal's head will happily eat hot dogs, Bologna 'sausage' or 'chicken' nuggets. These products regularly contain so-called 'mechanically recovered meat'. In this process, the (post-butchered) animal carcass, head and all, is squeezed under high pressure through a kind of sieve to remove any flesh that the butcher's knife has missed. The resulting paste is known appetisingly as 'white slime'.

However, accepting the reality of killing for meat doesn't mean that it's easy to do – and someone who is not comfortable or confident doing it is more likely to hesitate or make mistakes, which may cause unnecessary suffering to the animal. After a good deal of reflection and discussion we feel it would be unwise to offer a step-by-step guide to slaughtering rabbits or birds in this book. This is not out of squeamishness, or an unwillingness to engage with the issue, but rather because it's not something you can easily learn from a book. You should really attend one of the 'humane dispatch courses' that are available, or at a very minimum learn from the instructional videos on YouTube and elsewhere. The key is that animals are not unduly distressed before slaughter, and that they are slaughtered quickly and humanely. If you're not sure what you're doing, there's no guarantee you'll achieve either objective.

So, if you have never slaughtered a rabbit before, we strongly advise that you get some guidance from someone who has. The last thing you want to do is cause the animal extra suffering. Also make yourself aware of the current regulations governing slaughter for home consumption – they change from time to time. The most common home-slaughtering technique for rabbits is a firm blow to the base of the skull, with a heavy stick or other blunt object, stunning the animal. The rabbit's throat must then immediately be slit with a sharp knife to sever the two arteries, and the animal hung up by its back legs to bleed out. Some people remove the head completely rather than slitting the throat, but if you want to keep it for stock or soup – and we recommend that you do – it is easier to remove the fur if you leave it attached to the body.

As for squirrels, we're assuming that you are not raising your own. But if you set cage traps for them, you will also need to know how to humanely dispatch them. The recommended method is a firm blow to the head – but catching the animal and keeping it still can be tricky. Transfer the squirrel from the trap into a hessian sack, by tipping the trap or using sturdy gloves to avoid being bitten. Hold the squirrel, locate its head, and deliver a firm blow through the sack. You should then cut its throat, as with rabbits.

Butchering

Rabbits

If you get your rabbits from a butcher, they will normally come as a whole dressed carcass, or already jointed. Either way, you should try to get hold of the heart, liver and kidneys as well. They are very tasty, and are included in several of the recipes in this chapter. Get the head as well if you can. It's great for stock and gives a lovely rabbity richness to soups. Even the ears can be used (we provide a recipe on page 178).

If you catch or rear your own rabbits, or get them from a gamekeeper or farmer, you'll need to know how to butcher them yourself. This is really very easy. The steps are as follows. You need: a cleaver, kitchen scissors (or poultry shears) and a sharp utility or boning knife.

1. Starting with a dead rabbit, you first need to skin and paunch it (remove the innards). This should be done as soon as possible to reduce the risk of contamination. It can help to spray the carcass with water to prevent fluff flying everywhere. Using kitchen scissors, cut off all four feet at the joint, being careful not to shatter the bone (which will leave little shards in the meat). Next, use a sharp knife to slit the skin across the back, at right angles to the backbone. Make sure you cut only the skin and not the muscle – it's helpful to pinch some of the skin up before cutting. The cut should be a couple of inches or so in length – enough to get your fingers under for the next stage. (Some people prefer to cut the skin in a different place, either along the belly or the inside of the back legs; it's really just a matter of personal preference.)

2. Hook a couple of fingers from each hand under the skin, and pull in opposite directions. The skin should detach fairly easily and neatly, like removing a pair of gloves. The rear half of the skin should just pull off the back legs. If the fluffy tail doesn't come off with it, you will need to snip that off. Then concentrate on the head end. Ease the front legs out of the skin, so that now the pelt is attached only to the head. Peel the skin from the head, using a small knife if necessary to help work it loose. Remove the head and neck and keep for soup or stock.

3. With the skin removed, you now need to paunch the rabbit. Make a small cut in the belly, being very careful not to cut any of the innards. With the knife blade pointing outwards, extend the cut the full length of the belly while lifting the membrane away from the innards with two fingers. Remove the innards from the carcass, being careful not to tear the bladder or gall bladder. Keep the heart, kidneys and liver wrapped in cling film – we include them in some of the recipes that follow, or you can cook them in a similar way to bird organs (see the **Giblets** chapter). Discard the rest of the innards. Rinse out the cavity. (Some people like to soak the carcass for a few minutes in one or two changes of ice water, to remove more blood and cool the flesh; this is particularly useful in a hot climate.)

4. Lastly, remove any inner skin membrane or 'silverskin' from the carcass, as this can be tough. It can usually be pulled or cut off fairly easily. You should also cut away any excess fat, which you will usually only find with domestic rabbits. The rabbit is now ready to be cooked whole, or jointed.

5. To joint, first remove the back legs, which constitute up to 40 per cent of the dressed weight of a rabbit, and trim any remaining membrane or 'silverskin'. Then remove the front legs, or 'shoulders', which detach easily and are much smaller. Next remove the two flaps of belly meat attached to the ribs. You are then left with the saddle. Remove the pelvis, and also snip off the ribs, all of which you can use for stock or soup. Remove any remaining 'silverskin' from the saddle. The rest of the saddle can be left whole (such as for roasting). It can be cut into three sections for recipes that call for even-sized rabbit pieces (for the recipes below that list a jointed rabbit, this is what we mean). Or, the two loins (the fillets and surrounding flesh) – which are small but very tender – can be removed from the backbone (as for the paella recipe).

Squirrels

Butchering squirrels is rather similar to rabbits, with a few quirks. For one thing, squirrel skin is a fair bit harder to remove than rabbit. First, cut off the paws and tail – as with rabbits, be careful not to shatter any bones. Then start the skinning process in the same way as for rabbits: pinch up some skin on the back, make a cut perpendicular to the backbone, and start pulling the skin in opposite directions. The trick is not to pull so hard that you tear the beast in two, but hard enough to separate the skin. You'll need some help from the point of a sharp knife to ease away the skin in some places.

With the skin removed, proceed to paunch the squirrel. As with rabbits, make an incision along the belly, being careful not to cut into the innards, then remove the innards. The heart, kidneys, and liver are tiny treats that you should keep (see the **Giblets** chapter for some inspiration – they can be cooked in the same way as the corresponding rabbit and bird organs). Rinse the carcass well.

Having paunched the squirrel, decide how you are going to joint the carcass. Nearly all the meat is on the back legs, with a small amount on the loins and front legs – but these tasty morsels are definitely satisfying to pick at. Unless the recipe calls for whole squirrel, we therefore recommend using the head, neck, ribs and pelvis for soup or stock, and keeping the back and front legs and saddle (with belly flaps) for eating. In the recipes that follow, 'jointed squirrel' refers to these pieces.

RECIPES

A note on rabbit sizes: rabbits come in a range of different sizes depending on age, season and whether they are wild or reared. The following recipes, unless otherwise specified, call for a large wild rabbit or a medium-sized reared rabbit, with a dressed (butchered) weight of around 1 – 1.2kg. If your rabbit is much smaller than that – which many wild rabbits are – then two rabbits can be used.

Basics for cooking rabbit and squirrel

There are two clichés about rabbit: it's 'tough and dry', and 'it tastes a bit like chicken'. In fact, rabbit tastes nothing like chicken, and neither does squirrel (which is to say, since the person throwing that particular insult is presumably using over-cooked breast as a comparison, they actually taste of something); and although it is true that these meats have little fat, and therefore a tendency to dry out, there's no reason why they should be tough or dry, if cooked in the right way. We show you how. The secrets of tender rabbit and squirrel are long, slow cooking in liquid or fat, or adding a protective layer of moisture or fat in some other way, such as by larding or barding, or regular basting.

All recipes serve 4 unless otherwise noted.

Confit Rabbit Leg

4 rabbit legs (about 800g) – the rest of the rabbit may be used for the hearty rabbit soup recipe below

duck fat or olive oil (about 1 litre)

For green salt:

salt, black peppercorns, bay leaf, thyme, flat-leaf parsley

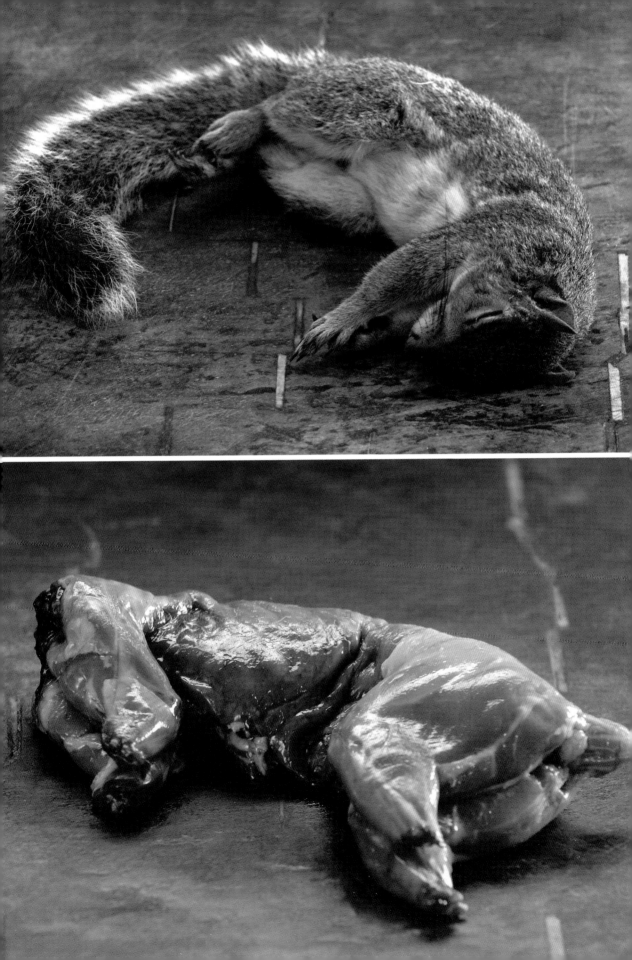

1. Weigh your rabbit legs. You need 5g of green salt per 100g of rabbit legs.

2. Make green salt by combining the following ingredients in a spice grinder or small food processor until well mixed and bright green:

  (a) 40g salt

  (b) 1.5g (half a teaspoon) black peppercorns

  (c) 1 bay leaf

  (d) 3g (about 3 sprigs) chopped thyme

  (e) 8g (about 3 sprigs) chopped parsley

3. Weigh out the appropriate amount of green salt and rub into the rabbit legs. Place in a tray in a single lay, cover, and refrigerate for 18 hours (too much longer and the legs will become over-salty). This salting stage improves the flavour and helps preserve the confit.

4. Pre-heat the oven to 90°C. Rinse the legs well under running water, then pat dry. Place in a heavy pot or casserole with lid and pour in enough fat/oil to cover. Place over medium heat until the fat is warm, then into the oven with the lid on for 10 hours. (Alternatively, cook sous vide for 8 hours at 82°C in 400g fat or oil.)

5. Carefully remove the legs from the fat (you can leave them to cool a bit first) and place in a storage container. Strain the fat over them, ensuring that they are completely covered; add more fat if not. Keep in the fridge for up to 2 weeks (longer storage is possible, but you will need to remove the meat juices from the fat before covering the legs).

6. To serve: remove the confit from the fridge a few hours early, so that the fat softens and the legs can be removed easily. Pre-heat the oven to 190°C. Heat an oven-proof frying pan over medium heat, and once it is hot add the rabbit legs. Fry for a couple of minutes on each side to lightly brown, drain any excess fat, then place in the oven for 5-10 minutes to heat through. Remove from the oven, drain the legs on paper towel, and serve with potato cubes sautéed in the excess fat and some wilted mangel-wurzel tops (recipe on page 202), spinach or Swiss chard.

Squirrel Rillettes

Confit two whole squirrels following the recipe for confit rabbit (up to stage 4), but reducing the salting time to 12 hours. Once cooled, remove from the fat, reserving 100g of fat. Remove the meat from the bones and shred it with your hands. You should have about 380g of meat. (If not, adjust the other quantities accordingly). Take half the meat, and stir in 40g Dijon mustard and plenty of freshly-ground black pepper. Gradually incorporate the reserved fat into the meat mixture – it will form a creamy emulsion. Stir in the rest of the meat and add salt and additional pepper to taste. Chill thoroughly to set. Remove from the refrigerator 30 minutes before serving, spread generously on toasted baguette slices, sprinkled with chopped toasted hazelnuts, and accompanied by a glass of champagne. An almost spiritual experience. (If you want a fully spiritual experience, caramelise the hazelnuts in maple syrup and butter and add a drop of Amaretto liqueur to your champagne...)

Hearty Rabbit Soup

This is a truly sensational soup that is definitely worth the effort to make. It's also a great way to make use of the rest of the rabbit if you like to confit the legs (we do).

1.2kg rabbit pieces, chopped into small chunks (any parts will do, especially ribs, pelvis, front legs and a head or two if you have any)

30g duck fat or olive oil

220g carrot, diced

220g leek, thinly sliced

1 shallot, finely chopped

2 litres chicken stock (preferably homemade)

1 clove garlic

1 bouquet garni (4 sprigs parsley, 2 sprigs thyme, 1 bay leaf, tied in muslin)

250ml double cream

salt and freshly-ground black pepper

chives, finely chopped

1. Heat the fat/oil in a large heavy-bottomed pan with lid. Gently sauté the carrot, leek and shallot, stirring occasionally, until softened (5-10 minutes).

2. Season the rabbit pieces with salt and pepper and add to the vegetables. Cover, and cook for 5 minutes. Remove the cover and cook for a further 10 minutes, turning the rabbit pieces occasionally until they are lightly browned all over.

3. Add the stock, garlic and bouquet garni and bring to a simmer. Cover the pan and simmer very gently for 5 hours.

4. Allow to cool a little then skim off as much of the fat as you can. Strain the liquid into a clean pan. Remove the bones from the strainer and discard, then press remaining solids through the fine blade of a food mill into the pan (if you don't have a food mill, purée the solids and press through a sieve).

5. Return to the boil and reduce to 1.2 litres. Add the cream, and season with salt and pepper to taste. Serve garnished with the chives.

Rabbit (or Squirrel) 'Provençal'

The combination of rabbit and onions is delicious (so delicious, here are two recipes, one French, one Greek).

1 large or 2 small rabbits (with liver and kidneys), jointed

125g butter

1 shallot, finely chopped

parsley, sage, rosemary and thyme

250ml red wine

a splash of red wine vinegar

sea salt

sugar

25–30 whole small peeled onions (the pickling – not the pickled – variety work well)

1. Add half the butter to a heavy saucepan and sauté the chopped shallot gently until soft.

2. Add the rabbit pieces to the pan, sprinkle with salt, pepper and herbs and brown all over; remove the rabbit from the pan.

3. Add the wine and vinegar, bring to the boil for 5 minutes, then add the rabbit back to the pan and simmer everything gently for an hour and a half, until the rabbit is tender.

4. While you're waiting for the rabbit to cook, add the other half of the butter to a large frying pan, add salt and sugar, and then the small onions all in one layer. Brown them quickly and add about 750ml of water; simmer the onions, covered, for about 15 minutes.

5. Remove the lid and cook the onions until they are tender and the liquid is reduced to a syrupy consistency (if the onions look like they're becoming too soft too soon, just remove them until you get the sauce as you want it and return them to the pan).

6. Remove the rabbit from the pan and reduce the wine and vinegar reduction until it too is syrupy, then add the baby onions and their cooking liquor to this. Return the rabbit to the saucepan.

7. Before serving, slice the rabbit liver and kidneys and cook in a little extra butter.

8. Serve the rabbit pieces with the small onions strewn all over with the rich sauce made from the wine reduction and the onion cooking liquor. Make sure everyone gets a little of the liver and kidney too.

This recipe is Provençal in origin. What follows is a Greek version of rabbit with onions, known as Kouneli Stifado.

Rabbit Stifado

Greek food is massively underrated. We're not sure why. One of the reasons, perhaps, is that what one tends to be offered in Greek restaurants outside Greece is such predictable fare. Also, Greek cuisine is, in the main, an exercise in simplicity, in which top quality ingredients are prepared with the minimum of fuss. In this regard it's unforgiving, since if you don't have the right ingredients, it simply won't work. You can hardly follow a recipe for a Greek tomato salad using the kind of Dutch billiard ball tomatoes we get in the UK and be surprised if the dish doesn't turn out the way It was when you tasted it in that seafront taverna in Naxos.

While they're not quite in the same league as wild rabbits in Greece, which feed on twigs of dried thyme and oregano and, to a more than negligible extent, marinate themselves from the inside out, wild rabbits in the UK are delicious too. This dish is one that does cross borders successfully.

1 rabbit, jointed

150ml extra virgin olive oil

250ml red wine

10 medium onions, cut into 4, but make sure you leave the small root piece in so that the pieces stay together while cooking

1 head garlic, peeled and roughly chopped

250ml of tomato passata or half a tube of tomato purée dissolved in enough warm water to make it the consistency of passata (that of a thick soup)

6 bay leaves

two 5cm long sticks of cinnamon
a little flour
salt and freshly-ground black pepper

1. Pre-heat the oven to 160°C.

2. Dredge the rabbit pieces in flour. Add the olive oil to a large ovenproof dish (or Dutch oven) and gently brown the rabbit pieces. Remove the rabbit to a plate.

3. Add the wine, scraping up all the bits on the bottom of the pan, then add the rabbit back to the pan with all the rest of the ingredients. Season with salt and lots (and lots) of black pepper.

4. Bring to the boil, cover with a lid and place in the pre-heated oven for at least 2 hours.

5. Remove from the oven and check the seasoning. Now turn up the oven a little, and return the pan to the oven without the lid. Cook for a further 20 minutes to half an hour.

When the dish is finished the sauce will have split slightly, and the juice that clings to the rabbit will be surrounded by a slick of ruby red olive oil. This is how it is supposed to be (and, to be honest, some of the versions we have had of this dish in Greece contain twice as much olive oil as the quantity we have suggested). Remember, olive oil represents up to half of the calorie intake of those Greeks who still enjoy what might be regarded as a 'traditional' Greek diet.

The cinnamon is very typical of Greek cooking, and the large quantity of bay leaves also. Greek dishes of oven-baked cockerel and lamb also feature these seasonings. Stifado is also prepared with hare (in which case marinate the meat in the wine for 8 hours or so) and, sometimes, beef. It's also delicious with squirrel (in which case, one per person).

Gibelotte

Gibelotte is another of those magic French words whose mere utterance causes saliva to run in a French mouth. My dictionary places its origin in the old French *gibelet* ('a dish of birds')... Today it means only rabbit and white wine stew.

R. Olney, *Simple French Cooking*, 1967.

Armed with the core techniques around which the above two recipes are constructed – which are not really so different to the core techniques in making a Daube de boeuf Bourguignon – you should find it fairly straightforward to cook up a Gibelotte. Olney, however, advises caution, and suggests cooking the rabbit in white wine and water first, and then preparing a garnish of baby onions separately (as in the Provençal recipe above). He is also quite strict on degreasing the sauce, so perhaps our stifado would not have found favour with him.

He suggests two deliciously different ways in which the final sauce of the Gibelotte can be enriched. Once the rabbit is cooking and resting, and you have reduced your sauce to the right consistency, either:

- Add a purée of sorrel cooked in butter and double cream in a ratio of 1 (sorrel and butter) to 2 (double cream). If you don't have sorrel, cook down some spinach in butter and, once it's mixed with the cream, add a generous splash of lemon juice.

- Thicken with two egg yolks mixed with 100ml double cream. This turns the Gibelotte into a fricassée.

Nearly twenty pages of *Simple French Cooking* are devoted to discussion of rabbit preparation and recipes (compared to five on pork, and ten on beef). If we've given you the bunny bug, we suggest you get a hold of a copy. It's a compelling, insightful volume.

Rabbit Ragù with Penne and Parmesan

This is our variation of the classic Tuscan dish *pappardelle con lepre*. Reassuringly rich, but surprisingly delicate flavours.

1 rabbit, jointed
180g onion, finely chopped
180g carrot, finely chopped
180g celery, finely chopped
120g bacon, diced
30g plain flour
salt and freshly-ground black pepper
50ml olive oil
250ml dry white wine
1 litre chicken stock (preferably homemade)
30g tomato purée
2 sprigs sage, chopped
1 stick cinnamon

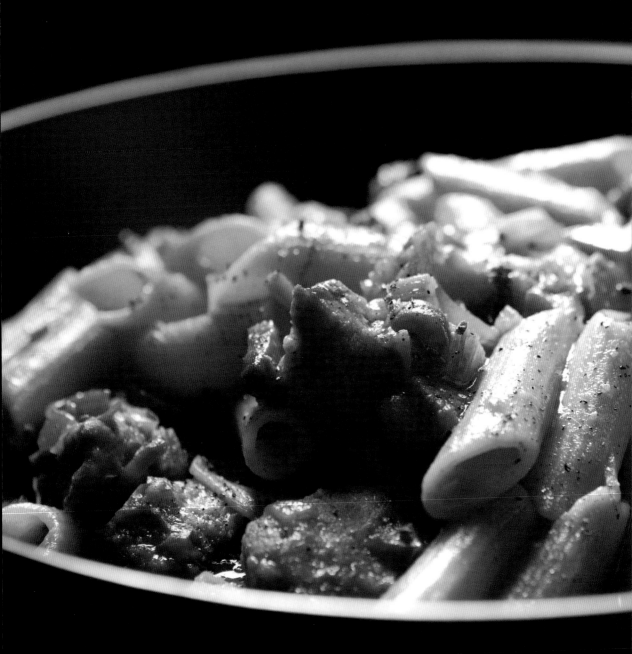

sherry vinegar
500g penne (or another dried pasta)
good quality parmesan cheese

1. Heat the oil in a large heavy-bottomed pan over medium-high heat. Sauté the onions, carrot and celery, stirring occasionally, until softened (5-10 minutes). Add the bacon and sauté for a further 5 minutes. Remove mixture and reserve.

2. Combine the flour with a teaspoon of salt and plenty of ground pepper on a large plate. Dredge the rabbit pieces in the mixture, then place the pan back over medium-high heat and brown the rabbit in batches (add a little extra oil if necessary). Remove and reserve.

3. Bring the wine to a boil, flame off the alcohol, then continue boiling for a couple more minutes, stirring to deglaze the pan. Add the rabbit and the reserved vegetable and bacon mixture. Add the chicken stock, tomato purée, sage and cinnamon. Reduce the heat and simmer, partially covered, for 45 minutes.

4. Remove the rabbit pieces and when cool enough to handle, pull the meat from the bones and shred coarsely by hand. Add the meat to the pan (discard the bones) and simmer uncovered for a further 45 minutes or until the sauce is thick. Discard the cinnamon stick. Stir a little sherry vinegar into the sauce.

5. Cook the pasta. Toss the sauce with the drained pasta, serve, and add a generous grating of parmesan and a few turns of black pepper.

Sauce au Vin de Médoc

I should... add that the name of this dish is not a printer's error, nor does it mean you throw away the meat and only eat the sauce; for, although the meat is cooked so slowly for so long that it practically is sauce, it is not uncommon in country districts of France to hear a stew of this kind referred to as *la sauce*.

Elizabeth David, *French Provincial Cooking*, 1967

1 rabbit, jointed
750g ox-cheek (or shin of beef) cut into large pieces
750g belly pork, skinned and cut into large pieces
olive oil
6 shallots, finely sliced
3 carrots (cut in to two or three pieces)

4 cloves garlic

1 bay leaf

a small sprig of thyme

a large bunch of parsley

a small amount of flour

750ml of wine

750ml of water

a little sugar

1 square of plain dark chocolate (75 per cent or more cocoa)

salt and freshly-ground black pepper

1. Heat the oil in a heavy saucepan with a tightly-fitting lid. Add the shallots and the carrots, sprinkle with salt and brown well.

2. Add the meat all in one go and brown well.

3. Add the garlic, herbs and a generous sprinkle of flour and mix well together.

4. Now add the wine, flame off the alcohol and let it boil vigorously for about 5 minutes.

5. Add the water, the sugar and square of chocolate. Simmer for about 3 hours, then allow to cool.

6. The next day, simmer again for 2 hours.

7. Before serving check the seasoning. If it is still a little sharp, add a little more salt and/or sugar.

As we mention in the recipe for Daube de boeuf Bourguignon, many stew recipes improve when they are cooled and reheated one, two or sometimes three times. It's something most modern cooks forget as part of their daily cooking life, but are reminded of each time someone says: 'Wow, this tastes even better than it did yesterday!' A little advanced thought is all that's required. Rowley Leigh suggests adding the offal that comes with the rabbit about an hour before the end of the cooking period. It's a lovely idea.

Lapin à la Fermière

This is an unusual cold rabbit dish from Elizabeth David's *Summer Cooking*. The original recipe calls for 750g of young broad beans, by which Elizabeth David means broad beans that are young enough for the pods to be cooked too; if you grow broad beans, then by all means do this, but for most of us, the broad beans we can get our hands on are always too old for the pods to be included.

1 rabbit, jointed

150g butter

500g shelled broad beans

1 leek, white and light green parts only, chopped

300g peas

2 potatoes, peeled and cut into 2 cm cubes

olive oil, lemon juice, garlic and lemon thyme for dressing

2 hard boiled eggs for garnish

salt and freshly-ground black pepper

1. Melt the butter in a pan and brown the well-seasoned rabbit pieces on each side.

2. Add all the vegetables, cover with water and simmer slowly for about 2 hours.

3. Remove the rabbit and dress while still hot with a vinaigrette made with 4 parts olive oil to 1 part lemon juice, a little garlic and some lemon thyme.

4. Remove the vegetables, keeping the cooking liquid for some soup, and sieve them (or blend them) to a firm purée.

5. Place the purée in the centre of a large serving platter and arrange the pieces of rabbit around it. Garnish with quarters of hard-boiled egg and serve with more vinaigrette

In winter, this dish can be served hot. Either keep the rabbit pieces warm while you're making the purée, or reheat them in a low oven (or, for that matter, in the pan in which they were originally cooked).

Rabbit Terrine

This is another cold rabbit dish. With the addition of some pork, rabbit makes a delicious terrine. It is much, much better if the meats are hand chopped rather than blitzed in a food processor.

1 rabbit, with offal

400g skinless belly pork

4 rashers of streaky bacon

75g butter

1 onion, finely chopped

3 cloves of garlic, finely chopped

a sprig of fresh thyme, leaves removed (oregano or marjoram works too)

1 egg

a shot of cognac or Armagnac

salt and freshly-ground black pepper

1. Pre-heat the oven to 160°C.

2. You will need to bone the rabbit. This is by no means as difficult as it sounds – the loin meat comes easily off the saddle and the rear legs have only a few bones, which are easily navigated. Also, since you're going to chop the meat finely, there's no pressure to take off neat fillets. You should get about 300g of meat from one reasonably sized rabbit.

3. Dice the rabbit (and its heart and liver) into very small pieces. Dice the belly pork and bacon to the same size. (The smaller the better – 1/2 cm dice is about what to aim for.)

4. Place all the meat on the biggest chopping board you have and with a heavy, sharp knife, chop it all together. After a few minutes you should have a nice homogenous mass.

5. Add the butter to a frying pan and sauté the onion and garlic gently for 10 minutes or so, until soft.

6. Put the cooked onion and garlic in a large mixing bowl and add the meat and all the rest of the ingredients. Season the mixture generously. (We find it useful to take a small ball of the terrine out with a teaspoon and cook it to check the seasoning. You might be surprised that the amount of salt, pepper and brandy you have added is nowhere near enough.)

7. Put the mixture in a 700ml capacity terrine and cover it with buttered greaseproof paper or foil and bake it in a bain-marie for up to 1.5 hours (or until the edges of the cooked mixture are coming away from the sides of the terrine). If you like, test the mixture by inserting a skewer, which should come out clean.

8. Leave the terrine to cool, then place it in the fridge weighted down with a few cans of baked beans.

9. Serve with cornichons or pickled walnuts.

Rabbit with Peanuts in Hot Bean Sauce

Very few people know more about Sichuan cuisine than Fuchsia Dunlop (and we include those people who live there). Ms Dunlop has studied in Chengdu, the capital of Sichuan Province, and speaks, reads and writes Mandarin. She is also a consultant to a number of Sichuanese restaurants in London. Her book *Sichuan Cookery* is a must for anyone interested in the food of that area.

1 rabbit, jointed

40g piece unpeeled fresh ginger

6 spring onions
(2 whole and 4 white parts only)

75g deep-fried or roasted peanuts

4 bird's eye chillies, thinly sliced

For the sauce:

peanut oil for frying

15ml fermented black beans, crushed with a spoon

50ml Sichuan chilli bean paste (Pi-Xian brand is good)

30ml light soy sauce

15ml white sugar

30ml sesame oil

Sichuan pepper, ground

1. Crush the ginger and the 2 whole spring onions with something heavy (a rolling pin is ideal) and place in a large pan of water. Bring this to the boil and add the rabbit pieces, return to the boil and skim.

2. Simmer over a low heat until the meat is just cooked, then remove the rabbit and allow to cool a little.

3. Remove all the meat from the bones.

4. To prepare the sauce, heat a large splash of peanut oil in a wok or frying pan over a medium flame until hot. Add the crushed fermented black beans and chilli bean paste. Stir-fry for 30 seconds – the oil will smell delicious and will have turned an appetising red colour, but make sure the mixture doesn't burn.

5. Transfer the sauce into a small bowl and combine with the soy sauce, sugar, sesame oil and a generous pinch of ground Sichuan pepper.

6. Cut the spring onion whites into quite thin slices. Place the rabbit meat, spring onions and peanuts on a shallow serving dish. Add the sauce and toss the mixture around so that everything is evenly coated. Top with the sliced chillies (you can use fewer if you like, but Sichuan food is famed for its pungency and spiciness and we like it that way).

Squirrel with Mustard

The combination of rabbit and mustard is a marriage made in heaven. The following recipe is an adaptation of the classic French recipe Lapin à la Moutarde, but uses squirrel instead. Feel free to use rabbit, of course, but if you do, you'll need to reduce the cooking time considerably – about an hour in the oven should do it. Squirrel has a uniquely fine texture, but it definitely takes longer to achieve the falling-off-the-bone tenderness that you're looking for. It also has a slightly more gamey flavour than rabbit, but is absolutely delicious. Indeed, in one of our houses squirrel is now the preferred ingredient for this dish. As we mentioned before, it's not the easiest meat to source, but Robert Gooch and his colleagues at the Wild Meat Company offer an excellent mail order service (wildmeat.co.uk) – or you could drive to Suffolk and pick it up yourself (they sell rabbit, hare and wild boar too).

You'll need one squirrel per person. There's not much meat apart from the back legs, but it's good fun picking the pieces up and biting off what there is, especially the loins. Squirrel liver is also delicious and your squirrel should come with this – you can chop it and add it at stage 5, or cook it using one of the liver recipes in the **Giblets** chapter.

4 squirrels, jointed

500ml dry cider

Dijon mustard

flour

butter

olive oil

4 shallots, finely chopped

4 cloves of garlic, finely chopped

100ml double cream

large bunch of parsley, leaves finely chopped

1. Pre-heat the oven to 150°C.

2. Reduce the cider by half over a high heat.

3. Smear the pieces of squirrel with a generous quantity of mustard and then dredge them in flour.

4. Brown the squirrel pieces in a mixture of butter and oil.

5. Remove the squirrel and add the shallots and garlic to the pan; soften them gently.

6. Once the shallots and garlic have softened, add the squirrel back to the pan with the reduced cider, cover, place in the oven and cook for 2 hours.

7. Remove the pan from the oven and test the squirrel for tenderness (by this time it should be starting to fall off the bone); check that there is enough liquid in the pan – if not, add some water or chicken (or squirrel) stock.

8. Add the double cream, and return to the oven for another hour.

9. Before serving add a generous handful of finely chopped parsley. A dollop of buttery mashed potato makes a nice accompaniment, and a slightly bitter salad too (think rocket or watercress).

Squirrel Stewed in Madeira

Here, as another variation on this theme, we re-create Brillat-Savarin's lost dish, mentioned in passing in *The Physiology of Taste* (he was too busy extolling the virtues of 'the four buxom daughters of Mr Bulow' to write down the recipe he developed on a visit to America).

4 squirrels, jointed

30g flour, well seasoned with salt and pepper

30g neutral oil

20g shallots, finely chopped

3 rashers of smoked streaky bacon, cut crossways into thin strips

250g mushrooms, sliced

150ml Madeira (dry Sercial type)

250ml squirrel, rabbit or chicken stock

a few sprigs of thyme

chopped parsley

1. Pre-heat the oven to 150°C.

2. Dust the squirrel pieces in the seasoned flour. Heat the oil in a Dutch oven or flameproof dish over high heat and brown the squirrel pieces in batches until golden-brown. Remove and reserve.

3. Gently sauté the shallots in the hot oil until soft. Add the bacon and sauté until just browned. Then add the mushrooms and cook until very soft and all the liquid has evaporated. Add the Madeira and bring to a boil. Flame off the alcohol, then add the stock and bring back to a simmer.

4. Add the squirrel pieces and thyme to the dish, cover and place in the oven. Cook for around 3 hours until completely tender, stirring occasionally.

5. Serve, topped with chopped parsley and maybe some wild rice or boiled new potatoes on the side.

Ice-filtered Squirrel Consommé

The perfect way to bring out squirrel's subtle gaminess, this consommé is clear as a crystal, and incredibly easy to get right. A pressure cooker makes things even easier. The chicken feet are important as they provide the gelatine that is crucial for the ice-filtering stage. Make this a couple of days ahead to allow the ice filtering to work its magic. The recipe also works well with rabbit.

Stock:

800g beef shank

500g chicken feet

4 whole squirrels (about 1.2kg)
(if possible include the kidneys – browned first – and heads)

100g carrot, finely diced

100g leeks, thinly sliced

60g fennel sprigs

60g spring onions

200ml white wine

100ml Noilly Prat (or other dry vermouth)

Aromatics:

2 whole star anise

2 cm piece of cinnamon stick

1 teaspoon black peppercorns

1 bay leaf

1 sprig thyme

1 small sprig rosemary

10g spring onions

For garnish:

chopped chives

1. Put half of the stock ingredients in a pressure cooker with 1.5 litres of water and cook at full pressure for 1 hour.

2. Strain, discard the solids and return the liquid to the pressure cooker with the other half of the stock ingredients (do not add more water), at full pressure for another 1 hour.

3. Strain again, discard the solids, and bring the liquid to a simmer. Remove from the heat, then add the aromatics and allow to infuse – off the heat – for 10 minutes. Remove the aromatics.

4. Pour into a large, flat-bottomed container and, when cool, put in the fridge until gelled. Transfer to the freezer.

5. Once frozen solid, dip the container into a sink of hot water to loosen the block. Lay a piece of muslin over a wire rack at least as large as the block, and place the block on top of the muslin. Place the rack over a tray and put into the fridge to defrost. As the block slowly melts, the gelatine will act as a filter, allowing a flavourful but perfectly clear consommé to drip into the tray. This will take about 24–48 hours, depending on the temperature of your fridge and dimensions of the block. (You can speed things up if you freeze into multiple smaller blocks.)

6. When ready to eat, reheat the consommé and add salt to taste. Serve in warm consommé bowls, with chopped chives on the side.

Ice-filtering is a great way to make a fool-proof and startlingly clear consommé. The only downside compared with the traditional approach is that the gelatine is removed in the filtration process, giving it a less rich mouthfeel. We think this works just fine for squirrel consommé, but if you prefer you can always add gelatine at stage 6 (about 10g/four sheets of leaf gelatine per litre).

Rabbit Burger

Rabbit makes a fantastic light and tasty burger, with some pork belly to add another layer of flavour as well as fat (rabbit is very lean).

900g rabbit mince (coarse grind)
300g minced pork belly (coarse grind)
1 medium onion, finely chopped
9g fine sea salt
3 egg yolks (optional; they add richness)
1 tablespoon finely chopped fresh herbs
(a mixture of oregano, thyme and sage is perfect)
neutral oil for frying

1. Mix all the ingredients together with your hands, then form into eight patties. Wrap in cling film and refrigerate for 30 minutes to an hour. This stage is important to allow the salt to begin binding the meat proteins, producing a cohesive burger; leave it too long, however, and the texture will become rubbery.

2. Heat a good glug of oil in a heavy-bottomed frying pan until very hot but not smoking, then reduce the heat to medium. Fry the patties in batches that will easily fit in the pan without touching. Fry for about 8 minutes, flipping the patties every minute until cooked through. Remove to drain on paper towels.

3. Serve with the normal burger accompaniments, definitely including mustard.

Spiced Squirrel Popcorn

A quick, tasty beer snack courtesy of 'wild gourmet' Thomasina Miers.

A note on the spices: some people call for dry roasting spices before grinding them. There is no question that this alters the flavour, in complex ways. But we don't think you should toast all spices, all the time; it depends on the spice and on the recipe. Here, we prefer raw spices.

2 squirrels, meat removed and cut into thin strips
15ml soy sauce
flour
neutral oil for frying

Seasoning:

1 teaspoon fennel seeds

1 teaspoon allspice

1 blade of mace

70g fine sea salt

1 teaspoon finely chopped fresh herbs (oregano, thyme and sage)

1. To make the seasoning, grind the spices to a fine powder in a spice grinder (or pestle and mortar). Mix with the salt and herbs.

2. Mix together the meat and soy sauce, then dredge each piece in flour.

3. Deep fry the squirrel in small batches until crispy and golden-brown, making sure the oil remains hot, but not smoking. Drain on kitchen paper, then sprinkle with the seasoning.

Brunswick Stew

We reproduce here the first known printed recipe of this squirrel-and-butterbean stew from the southern US, from Marion Harland's 1871 book of recipes, *Common Sense in the Household*. The stew is named after Brunswick County, Virginia where Mrs Harland reports that it 'is a famous dish – or was – at the political and social picnics known as barbecues'. Brunswick Stew is still popular, but nowadays is all too often made with chicken. We have reproduced it essentially unchanged, other than converting to metric measures.

2 squirrels – 3, if small

800g tomatoes, peeled and sliced

400g butter (Lima) beans

6 potatoes, parboiled and sliced

6 ears of green [young] corn cut from the cob

225g butter

225g fat salt pork or bacon

1 teaspoonful ground black pepper

half a teaspoonful cayenne

3.8 litres water

15g salt

8g white sugar

1 onion, finely chopped

Put the water with the salt in it, and boil 5 minutes. Put in the onion, beans, corn, pork or bacon cut into shreds, potatoes, pepper, and the squirrels, which must first be cut into joints and laid in cold salt water to draw out the blood. Cover closely and stew 2 1/2 hours very slowly, stirring frequently from the bottom. Then add the tomatoes and sugar, and stew an hour longer. Around 10 minutes before you take it from the fire, add the butter, cut into bits the size of a walnut, rolled in flour. Give a final boil, taste to see that it is seasoned to your liking, and turn into a soup tureen. It is eaten from soup plates.

Deep-fried Rabbit Ears

It may sound weird or downright unpalatable, but this recipe was developed by Ferran Adrià for his world famous restaurant El Bulli, and published in *El Bulli 2003–2004*. They are surprisingly, amazingly delicious – like delicate, super crunchy pork scratchings. Kudos also to the *Hungry in Hogtown* blog for tackling this one step-by-step at home. Here's our version.

Note: You can make the herb powders by blitzing commercial dried herbs in a spice grinder, but it's even better to use fresh herbs that you've dried yourself. They don't need to be ground to a uniformly fine powder – a mixture of sizes works well.

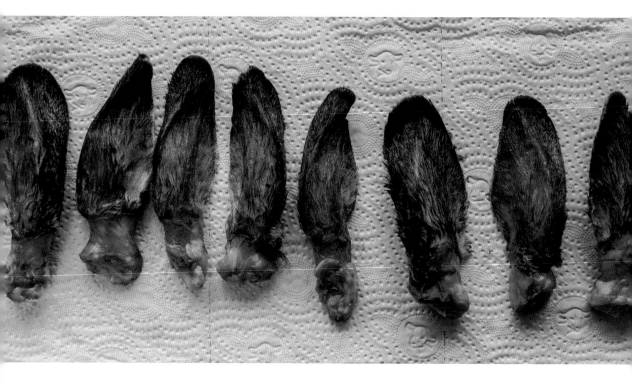

8 rabbit ears
neutral oil for deep-frying
a clove of garlic, cut in half
fleur de sel or Maldon salt
thyme and rosemary powder

1. Soak the ears in two changes of cold, lightly salted water for 12–24 hours to clean them of any blood residue. (Keep them in the fridge while soaking.)

2. Blanch the ears for one minute in boiling water. Remove the ears, refill the pot with clean water, and bring back to the boil. Add the ears and simmer for 30 minutes.

3. Remove the ears, and while still hot, rub off the fur and any blood vessels (some of these may need to be scraped away with a knife).

4. Place the ears on a wire rack in the fridge to dry (or if you want to do it more quickly, put them in a very low oven). They do not need to be completely dehydrated, but the drier they are, the less they will spit when you fry them.

5. Deep-fry the ears in hot (180°C) oil until crispy, taking care to use a splatter guard. (The residual moisture in the ears will cause them to spit a lot, and their funnel shape can shoot spurts of boiling oil a fair distance.)

6. Remove the ears and drain on paper towels. When cool enough to handle, rub the ears with the cut side of the halved garlic clove. Sprinkle with the salt, crushed a little if the flakes are large. Dust with some powdered herbs and serve.

Rabbit Paella

A Valencian speciality, originally made with water vole. It looks fabulous and tastes even better. Snails are traditional, but prawns do very nicely too. This will serve four very hungry people.

2 rabbits (with liver and kidneys if possible)

For rabbit stock:

2 litres water
100g carrots, roughly chopped
100g leeks, roughly chopped
100g onions, roughly chopped

1 bay leaf

3 sprigs thyme

small bunch parsley, stalks only (leaves reserved for garnish)

For paella:

90ml olive oil

200g red onion, finely chopped

1 red pepper, deseeded and cut into thin strips

3 cloves garlic, finely chopped

30g tomato purée

half a teaspoon smoked paprika

pinch of saffron threads

360g paella rice (or Arborio), rinsed

50ml Noilly Prat (or other dry vermouth)

12 live mussels, scrubbed clean

12 raw shelled snails (alternatively, 12 uncooked prawns in shells)

flat-leaf parsley leaves, chopped (reserved from stock ingredients, above)

salt and freshly-ground black pepper

1. Remove the back legs from the rabbits, aiming to include as much meat as possible. Remove the two loins from the saddle, and cut each into three pieces. Reserve the back legs and loin pieces for the paella. Use the rest of the rabbits for the stock.

2. Make a rabbit stock as follows. Cut the remaining parts of the rabbits into several pieces and place in a large pan. Add the liver and kidneys, or a small quantity of chicken giblets if you don't have them. Add the water, bring to a simmer and skim. Add the rest of the stock ingredients and simmer for 45 minutes, skimming regularly. Remove from the heat and pass the liquid through a fine sieve into another container, leaving behind any solids or very cloudy liquid at the bottom of the stock pan. You should have about 1.8 litres of stock. You will need 600ml for this recipe; the remainder can be frozen and used the next time you make paella, or for rabbit ragù or squirrel stewed in Madeira.

3. Set the oven to 200°C to pre-heat.

4. Heat the oil in a paella pan or ovenproof sauté pan, until very hot. Season the rabbit legs with plenty of salt and pepper and brown well on both sides, then remove and reserve.

5. Reduce the heat and add the onion and pepper to the same oil. Sauté until soft, about 8 minutes, then add the garlic and sauté for a couple more minutes. Add the tomato purée and cook for a couple of minutes more, then stir in the paprika, saffron and rice.

6. Next put the browned rabbit legs and the pieces of rabbit loin in the pan and cook for a minute or two. Pour over 600ml of the rabbit stock and the vermouth. Season with salt and black pepper.

7. Bring back to a simmer, remove from the heat and cover with foil or a tight-fitting lid. Place in the oven and cook for 10 minutes.

8. Remove the pan and bury the mussels and snails (or prawns) in the rice. Cover and return to the oven for a further 10–15 minutes, until most of the liquid has been absorbed and the rice is al dente (if it looks like the liquid will be absorbed earlier than this, add a little more stock). Then turn off the oven and leave the pan to rest in the warm oven for a further 5 minutes or so until the remainder of the liquid has been absorbed but the rice is still moist – the consistency should be a little firmer than a risotto, but not dry and fluffy like a pilaf.

9. Serve, garnished with parsley.

Numerous variations on this dish are possible. You can replace some of the stock with white wine (say, 150ml). Rosemary works well instead of thyme. Any kind of seafood can be added – clams, cockles, scallops or whelks (our favourite). For a special occasion, chunks of lobster meat or whole langoustines are great. Baby squid work well, and even better would be chunks of octopus arm – either pre-cooked in a pressure cooker (see page 30) with the liquor added to the stock, or semi-dried and grilled (page 33) and stirred into the final dish. Slices of chorizo, browned with the meat, add another layer of flavour. The possibilities are endless – no need to follow this recipe exactly, see what's available and make it your own.

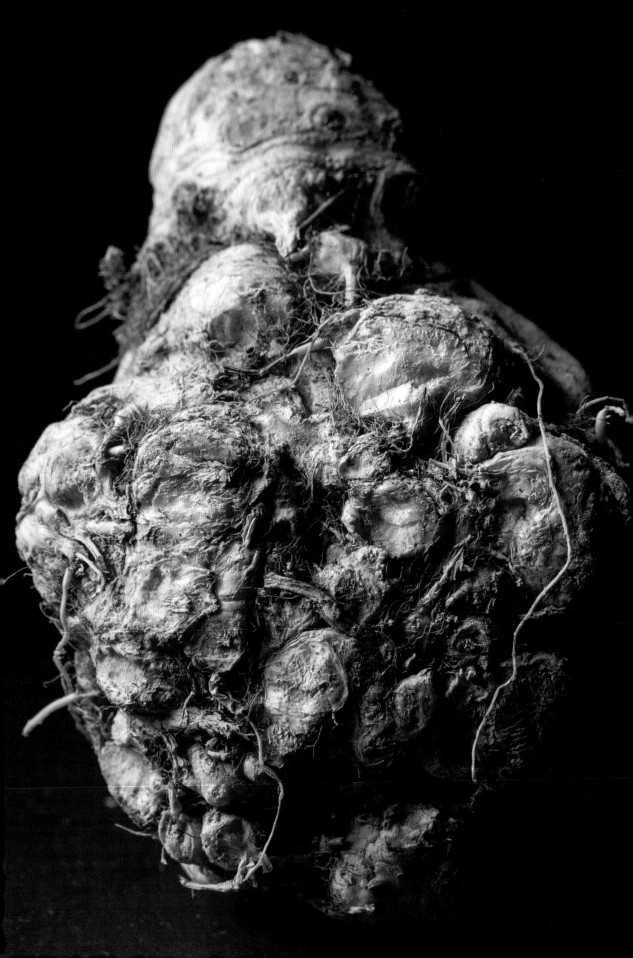

6. UGLY VEG

Beet that!

The famed British cavalry officer John Le Marchant (1766–1812) saw action in the disastrous Flanders Campaign during the French Revolutionary Wars. He was greatly impressed by the Austrians, who he fought alongside, and seemed to take to heart their view that British swordsmanship was like 'someone chopping wood'. He designed a new sabre, and in 1796 completed a detailed training manual on mounted swordsmanship, which was adopted by the army as its standard Rules and Regulations of the Sword Exercise of the Cavalry.

One of the most devastating of sword moves in a skilled hand is the 'drawing cut', where the length of the blade is pulled back once the target has been struck. This 'has the additional advantage of deepening the wound and of cutting into the bone', according to Richard Burton's *The Book of the Sword*. But getting just the right action and force to penetrate hard flesh was a little more difficult than standard fencing. The solution? A large and much-maligned root vegetable called the mangel-wurzel. Placed on a table, it rolled around like a real victim, and replicated pretty well the power and technique needed to separate head from shoulders. (You can substitute a turnip at a pinch.)

We're all in favour of slicing up mangel-wurzels with large blades. But we prefer to do so in the pursuit of a different calling: Mangel-Wurzel Confit (recipe on page 202).

Mangel-wurzel. Celeriac. Jerusalem artichoke. Hamburg parsley. Salsify. Slow-cooked, roasted, sliced raw in salads or cooked in a variety of different ways, these ugly vegetables make up for in flavour what they lack in outward appearance. We provide the stories behind a range of somewhat obscure but tasty vegetables and explore the changing role of the root vegetable in European cuisines.

We also spare a thought for all those misshapen fruit and vegetables that are currently discarded in order that our supermarket shelves can be filled with shiny, homogeneous, and tasteless things.

There seems to us to be something deeply wrong with buying imported asparagus in December, or tiny string beans in the depths of Winter. It is undeniable that one of the reasons those tiny, film-wrapped trays of asparagus or beans or gleaming 'tenderstem' broccoli or mangetouts sell so well is the misperception that because they look attractive they must therefore be delicious and healthy in a way that our own home-grown root vegetables are not. This chapter aims to redress the balance.

Beta vulgaris vulgaris

> The beet was Rasputin's favourite vegetable. You could see it in his eyes.
>
> In Europe there is grown widely a large beet they call the mangel-wurzel. Perhaps it is mangel-wurzel that we see in Rasputin. Certainly there is mangel-wurzel in the music of Wagner...
>
> Tom Robbins, *Jitterbug Perfume*

Beta vulgaris vulgaris – so vulgar they named it twice. The *vulgaris* subspecies of the common beet is indeed everywhere, the most grown of all beets. The beetroot (garden beet), chard (silverbeet), mangel-wurzel (mangold) and sugar beet are all cultivars of this same subspecies. And all of them taste great – with the exception of sugar beet, which was developed not for eating but as a source of sugar for refining (and which one of our mothers, who tried to eat one in a field during the War, assures us was foul). Apart from sugar cane, sugar beet is the only source of sucrose, accounting for about a quarter of global supply.

In many ways, the mangel-wurzel is the most amazing of them all. Its leaves and stems have a fantastic flavour, easily the equal of Swiss chard. Its root, while not as lascivious as a deep red beetroot, can be just as luscious – and even sweeter (it has a sugar content of about 8 per cent, compared to just 3 per cent for regular beetroot). And it doesn't threaten to stain your hands and chopping board and everything else within a six foot radius an indelible red. According to seventeenth-century herbalist Nicholas Culpeper, it grows in just about any soil and is able 'to constantly thrive, and to produce a very great crop, even when other kinds of roots and vegetables fail, and when there is a general scarcity of forage'. (This comes from his book with the wonderful title: *Culpeper's Complete Herbal, Wherein Several Hundred Herbs, With a Display of Their Medicinal and Occult Properties, are Physically Applied to the Cure of all Disorders Incident to Mankind*). One thing Culpeper got wrong was the etymology. He called mangel-wurzel the 'root of scarcity', from the German *mangel* ('scarce') and *wurzel* ('root'); he assumed this meant it was eaten in lean times when it was the only thing available. In fact, the English word is a corruption of the German *mangold*, which means 'beet', so the original *mangoldwurzel* literally meant 'beet root'.

Mangel-wurzel is widely grown in Britain. It is a staple of rural culture, giving rise to the children's-book scarecrow Worzel Gummidge (so named because his head was made of one) and the 'scrumpy and western' band The Wurzels ('I got 20 acres and you got 43 / Now I got a brand new combine harvester and I'll give you the key'). In Somerset, Punkie Night is celebrated on the last Thursday of October, with children – led by a Punkie King and Punkie Queen – carrying around jack o'lanterns made of hollowed-out mangel-wurzels ('punkies') and playing a version of trick-or-treat. Some country folk make cheap beer (recipe on page 203) or moonshine from them, something their high sugar content makes them perfect for.

Mangel-wurzels are everywhere, but no one thinks of eating them. Diane Morgan's excellent 'definitive compendium' *Roots* doesn't mention them. Even at the Mangold Hurl, an annual October gathering in the West Country described as 'what you get if you mix *boules* and strong cider' and 'possibly the greatest of the vegetable throwing events', there are no mangold snacks available. The website of the Mangold Hurling Association, an otherwise staid compendium of rules and gameplay, has a very small collection of satirical recipes. The event itself is surely one of the more bizarre of the English sports, claiming to have an ancient history. According to the rules – which are suspiciously similar to those of the spoof sport of 'haggis hurling', invented in the 1970s – competitors take it in turns to hurl mangel-wurzels, grasped by the leafy top, at a pre-placed 'Norman' (a larger mangel-wurzel with the top removed). The competitor whose mangold is closest to the Norman is crowned the Mangold King – with a wreath of mangold leaves, naturally.

Back in the real world, mangel-wurzels have appeared in literature, including a mention in W. Somerset Maugham's *Of Human Bondage*, albeit as a way of telling if someone knew country life. They were also mentioned prominently in George Orwell's *Animal Farm*, appearing in the revolutionary song 'Beasts of England' for whom the revolution would bring 'clover, beans and mangel-wurzel'.

Mangel-wurzels are indeed mainly grown as a winter feed for cattle, and perhaps it is this, together with their strange name, that makes them an object of derision rather than culinary desire. But if picked young, before they get too big and fibrous, they taste great.

There are many other ugly vegetables, particularly root vegetables, that used to be popular – or, in many cases, were the only option available in the long winter months – but that have fallen into obscurity as all kinds of superficially prettier produce have become available all year round. Here we look at some of our favourites.

The Beet Generation

Many of the roots in this chapter will keep for a long time – in some cases, up to six months in ideal conditions. And indeed, one of the traditional reasons for growing root vegetables has been to have a stock of nutritious food to last through the winter. So if you grow your own, and have a root cellar or other place where they will keep well, you can enjoy them over an extended period. But just because they can be kept for a long time doesn't necessarily mean that they should be. Like other vegetables, they are mostly at their best when fresh, losing some of their zing over time. Fresh mangel-wurzel is much better. Salsify and burdock become limp and less exciting if stored for more than a day or two. Celeriac loses a lot of that powerful celery flavour that is so appealing, and its delightful fresh crunch; Jerusalem artichokes fare much the same. And kohlrabi is so much better if you can pick it, peel it, and use it immediately – with a sweet, apple-like soul that soon departs the body. So if you are buying your roots, try to get the freshest ones you can, and eat them up quickly.

MANGEL-WURZEL

We think the mangel-wurzel is ripe for a makeover. 'Mangold' sounds much better, suggestive of their golden hue. Some people call them 'golden beets', although that can get confusing, because there are also red-skinned and orange-skinned varieties, and there are yellow-gold cultivars of regular beetroot. But then, maybe mangel-wurzel isn't all that bad a name. According to Culpeper, an alternative name is 'dick wurzel'; just imagine the derision if that had caught on.

It's almost impossible to find mangel-wurzels in shops, but you can get some from a friendly farmer, or better still it is very easy to grow your own. Pick them on the young side, when the tops are still verdant and tender – and you can harvest some of the leaves before you pull the root. Once the root is pulled, eat it within a day or two, while still fresh. We hope that they start making an appearance at farmers' markets, and from there to the high street.

JERUSALEM ARTICHOKE (SUNCHOKE)

The Jerusalem artichoke (*Helianthus tuberosus*) is not an artichoke and has nothing to do with Jerusalem. But don't let the obscurity of the name put you off – they taste absolutely fabulous, whether raw, roasted, steamed, or as a soup. They are fairly widely available, and we urge you to make these tubers a regular part of your cooking.

Now, if you're a farmer in the Midwest of the United States, you may be getting rather suspicious at this point. You see, the Jerusalem artichoke was the basis for what must be one of the most unlikely pyramid schemes ever hatched. In the early 1980s, in the wake of the 1979 oil crisis, the US government was exploring new ways of making biofuel for vehicles. A trio of conmen got in on the act, promoting the Jerusalem artichoke as a profitable cash crop for farmers: the plant is an excellent source of ethanol, they said, and a valuable sweetening agent could also be obtained as a by-product. Best of all, the plant grew well on marginal soils with minimal agricultural inputs. This was mostly true, but there was no established market; the promoters of the crop were simply after a quick buck. In a classic pyramid scheme, first-year growers were enlisted to convince other farmers to participate, with most of the initial crops used to produce seeds to sell to farmers who joined later. The company established by the conmen sold $25 million worth of seeds to Midwestern farmers. When the time came for farmers to begin selling their crops, however, no agri-business companies were interested, resulting in thousands of acres of useless produce. At trial one of the conmen, a devout Christian, had a ready explanation: 'It was Satan who stopped the Jerusalem artichoke,' he said, 'because of all the good it would do.'

He may have been on to something. There is a vaguely devilish character to the Jerusalem artichoke, and we're not talking about its tempting earthiness. We think John Goodyer put it best, in his entry in the 1633 revision of Gerard's *Herball*:

In my judgement, which way soever they be dressed and eaten, they stir up and cause a filthie loathsome stinking wind within the body, thereby causing the belly to be much pained and tormented, and are a meat more fit for swine than man…

And while we strongly dispute the conclusion that they are only fit for swine, there's no denying their propensity to cause flatulence in some people. There is, however, a scientific explanation. Jerusalem artichokes store energy in the form of inulin, a fructose polymer that humans lack the enzymes to digest (inulin also occurs in burdock, dandelion, chicory and many other plants). Beneficial bacteria living in our colons can break down inulin, but produce hydrogen and carbon dioxide gases as they do so, which is where the flatulence comes from. Excessive inulin consumption can also cause diarrhoea, abdominal pain and bloating – but the effects are very variable across individuals, depending on the particular microflora present in their gut, which is in turn influenced by how much inulin they have eaten in the past. In short, the more you eat at one sitting, the more noticeable the effects; but the more you eat over time, the more tolerant you will become.

Eat more Jerusalem artichoke!

The plant is actually a species of sunflower native to North America (and therefore is related – but only distantly – to the globe artichoke). Its name is an English corruption of the Italian word *girasole*, which means 'sunflower'; girasole artichoke thus became Jerusalem artichoke. The 'artichoke' part comes from the fact that the tubers taste vaguely like globe artichokes – something pointed out by the seventeenth-century explorer Samuel de Champlain when he sent the first samples of the plant back to his native France (by this time, it was already known in Italy):

Sieur de Poutrincourt landed [at Gloucester Bay, Cape Ann] with eight or ten of our company. We saw some very fine grapes just ripe, Brazilian peas, pumpkins, squashes, and very good roots, which the savages cultivate, having a taste similar to that of chards [blanched shoots of globe artichoke or salsify]. They made us presents of some of these, in exchange for little trifles which we gave them.

Voyages of Samuel de Champlain 1604-1618

Jerusalem artichokes are very easy to grow – so easy, that the biggest problem tends to be stopping them from spreading once they've established themselves. The best results – crisp and flavourful – require cool soil temperatures. Thus, although they can be grown and harvested over much of the year, it is best to harvest or buy them from late autumn to mid-winter. The colder the area you live in, the earlier they should be harvested – ideally after the first hard frost in cold areas, and later into the winter in milder regions.

The later they are left, the larger the tubers will become. And while they can be stored in a cool root cellar, they are best eaten soon after harvesting, so we recommend that you dig them up as you need them and leave the ones you don't need to keep growing.

Salsify

Salsify root is also known as oyster vegetable or oyster plant, in reference to its somewhat bitter but wonderfully delicate salty and rather oyster-like flavour – so much so that Dorothy Hartley assures us in *Food in England* that it is so realistic that 'it takes in the cat!'. We love it, but popular opinion appears remarkably divided on whether it really does taste like oyster, and whether it's any good – this may be partly due to variation in flavour and quality depending on the cultivar, how it was grown and when it was harvested. But we urge you to get hold of some and give it a try.

Cooking Salsify

Cut the scraped or peeled salsify into 3 inch lengths, slicing the thicker parts into two or four lengthways so they are all about the same thickness. Keep the pieces in acidulated water (that is, water with about 7ml lemon juice or vinegar added per litre) until you are ready. Cook in a large pot of salted water at a rolling boil (the more water, the less the temperature drops when you add the salsify – a good principle for boiling any vegetable). Start checking doneness after 15–20 minutes, and cook until tender but still slightly firm.

True salsify (*Tragopogon porrifolius*) has a long, thin root – often together with some smaller rootlets – and has white skin. *Tragopogon* is the Greek for 'goat's beard', an alternative name for the plant. Black salsify (*Scorzonera hispanica*) has a similarly long root, with black skin and an absence of rootlets, making it easier to peel. Although different species, they are both members of the huge sunflower family and taste similar; black salsify tends to have less of the characteristic oyster flavour. Jerusalem artichoke is a member of the same family, as is burdock.

Two great authorities diverge on how long salsify is best cooked for. *Larousse Gastronomique* suggests 60–90 minutes 'according to the quality of the vegetable' while Elizabeth David in *French Provincial Cooking* recommends 20–25 minutes, adding that 'most cooks say 40 minutes: it is too long'. We tend more towards Elizabeth David's timing, but different cultivars as well as individual roots are very variable (and we're not convinced that white and black salsify cook exactly the same). As the roots get older, and larger, they become tougher and less palatable. It is best to buy and cook salsify fresh, when the roots are firm and stiff.

Burdock root

Burdock is the common name for plants in the genus *Arctium*, part of the large sunflower family (Asteraceae) that also includes dandelion, Jerusalem artichoke, lettuce, and salsify, along with more than 23,000 other species. Its prickly seeds were the inspiration for Velcro, and its root has been used in Chinese medicine since ancient times. But the young roots were also popular in cooking due to their appealing texture and flavour – crunchy, slightly sweet, and somewhat earthy. They are long, brown and slender in appearance. Older roots can tend to become fibrous and tough.

Kilim rugs, particularly those from Turkey, often contain *pitrak* or stylised burdock motifs which are believed to ward off the evil eye – a curse cast by a malevolent glare. Nicholas Culpeper, in his *Herbal*, ascribes it great medicinal powers:

> A drachm of the roots, taken with pine kernels, helpeth them that spit foul, mattery, and bloody phlegm; the leaves applied to the places troubled with the shrinking of the sinews or arteries, give much ease; the juice of the leaves, or rather the roots themselves, given to drink with old wine, doth wonderfully help the bitings of serpents; and the root beaten with a little salt, and laid on the place, suddenly easeth the pain thereof, and helpeth those that are bit by a mad dog...

In the *Encyclopaedia Perthensis* of 1816, it was cited as a cure for a completely different affliction, baldness, in what sounds like the beginning of a recipe for wine braised root vegetables (recipe, page 199):

> Where the baldness is total, a quantity of the finest burdock roots are to be bruised in a marble mortar, and then boiled in white wine, until there remains only as much as will cover them. This liquor, carefully strained off, is said to cure baldness, by washing the head every night with some of it warm.

Frankly, it's likely to be about as effective as modern baldness remedies. Which means that you can rub one of those into your scalp instead, or nothing at all, and rather eat the braised burdock, with some celeriac and a sprig of rosemary.

Burdock is a fairly common wild plant that is popular with foragers, and is a local delicacy in some places – including the South of France where the pleasantly bitter young stems and young leaves are added to soups or served braised. But it never really made it into mainstream Western cooking. More recently, though, it has gained some popularity as part of macrobiotic diets – advocated for their purported health benefits.

Many people in the United Kingdom will have come across it in a drink called 'dandelion and burdock', a kind of root beer that has been consumed since the middle ages and is still produced commercially. Originally it was a lightly alcoholic drink made from fermented dandelion and burdock roots. However, like ginger beer it evolved to become a soft drink – usually now using artificial flavours with no actual dandelion or burdock extracts.

Preparing burdock

To prepare, carefully scrub the roots to clean them and remove any rootlets. Do not peel them, as the skin is thin, tender and has the best flavour. Cut them into convenient lengths or into a julienne. Like salsify and Jerusalem artichoke, they will quickly discolour in air, so hold them in acidulated water. In fact, a 15–30 minute soak in cold water is generally recommended, as burdock root can otherwise have a muddy taste; it also reduces the bitterness. As with other roots, they can be stored, but are best kept a little moist and eaten while still firm. A freshly-pulled root definitely tastes best.

Burdock is widely used in Japanese cooking, where it is known as *gobo* its culinary use is documented as far back as the tenth century. Mainly prized for its crunchy texture and ability to take on other flavours, as well as for its purported restorative properties, the young leaves are also sometimes eaten. It is traditionally cut into 'rolling wedges' (*ran-giri*), a series of diagonal slices where the root is rotated a quarter turn between cuts, resulting in small uneven pieces; or, into 'shavings' (*sasagaki*), as if you were sharpening a pencil with a penknife.

Burdock roots may be available in farmers' markets or health-food shops, but it's not generally that easy to find for sale in Western outlets. Its popularity in East Asian cooking, though, means that it should be available in Japanese and Korean shops. The wild plant is also so widespread that it's easy to obtain your own. But make sure you know what you are doing, or take advice from someone who does, and please don't confuse it with deadly nightshade root, which could be, well, deadly. Also be aware that the root is very long – up to a metre – and the plant often prefers stony soil – a combination that led one herbalist to describe it as 'a bitch to dig'. Choose those growing on damper, softer soil, and take a big spade.

Celeriac (celery root)

Celeriac is a variety of celery grown for its large root. (Strictly speaking, it's not a true root but rather another type of storage organ known as a hypocotyl or tuber.) Celery and celeriac derive from a wild plant called smallage (*Apium graveolens*) which grows in marshlands and coastal areas across Eurasia. It was known to the ancients as *selinon* or *helioselinon*, was mentioned by Hippocrates and Pliny, and described in Homer's *Odyssey* as part of a scene of bucolic bliss:

> There was a large fire burning on the hearth. One could smell from afar the fragrant odour of burning cedar and sandal wood. Calypso was busy at her loom, shooting her golden shuttle through the warp and singing beautifully. Round her cave was a thick wood of alder, poplar, and sweet smelling cypress trees. Therein were all kinds of great birds which had built their nests – owls, hawks, and chattering sea gulls whose business is in the waters. A vine loaded with grapes was trained and grew luxuriantly about the mouth of the cave. There were also four running rills of water in channels cut pretty close together. They were turned hither and thither to irrigate the beds of violets and luscious herbage, including smallage [wild celery], over which they flowed. Even a god could not help being charmed with such a lovely spot.

Smallage was used in medicine, but apparently not for cooking. It was only in the seventeenth century that it began to be cultivated for food, initially for its leaves which were used in soups, then for its stems and root. Two main types were developed: one with thickened stems and a small root, widely eaten now as celery. The first cultivars were described as having a very strong hot and bitter flavour, but continued cultivation led to larger, more tender stems with an increasingly mild flavour – probably through cross-breeding, growing it later in the season, and reducing the bitter taste by 'blanching' (banking up earth to deprive the stems of light). The second type of celery was developed for its large bulbous stem base (hypocotyl); the stems themselves remained small and tough like smallage.

One of the reasons the ancients had for not eating celery, apart from the excessively strong taste of the wild variety, is that it was associated with death, funerals and the underworld. Pliny states explicitly that it is only to be eaten at funeral banquets. The Isthmian Games of Ancient Greece, which Sisyphus reputedly instituted as funeral games in honour of a mythological wrestler, crowned the victors with a wreath of celery. Posterity does not record whether they were allowed to eat it.

So if smallage was associated with death, was not generally used in cooking, and was mostly reserved for medicinal purposes, why the specific reference to it in the *Odyssey*? The 'four running rills of water' certainly provide a very suitable habitat for wild celery. But there may have been another reason for choosing to single out this one plant from among the 'luscious herbage'. The curly leaves of wild celery apparently gave it the additional meaning of 'female pubic hair', according to Andrew Dalby's *Food in the Ancient World*. But we have no idea if Homer was making lewd references in the above passage, or if he was just a celery fan.

In fact, historians aren't totally sure exactly what the ancient Greeks and Romans meant by *selinon*. The normal translation is smallage, or wild celery, but the word appears to have also been used more-or-less interchangeably for parsley, which was considered a variant of celery. Modern classification has them in the same broad family (Apiacaea), but not more closely related than that.

Perhaps it was the pubic connotations that led to another reputed use of celery in the late middle ages: as an aphrodisiac. Local German names include *geilwurtz* ('horny herb') and *stehsalat* ('erection salad'), and according to a German medical handbook quoted in a modern anthology, the application was simple:

> Then if you want your wife to love you above all other men, take some celery juice crushed and blended with honey and apply it to the member and testicles, that will make her love none other above you.

> Marcel Cleene & Marie Lejeune,
> *Compendium of Symbolic and Ritual Plants in Europe*, 2002

If you do decide to smother yourself with honey and celery juice, we'd prefer you didn't mention that you got the idea from us.

Hamburg parsley (parsley root)

Hamburg parsley root is fantastic – savoury and assertive, with a great texture like celeriac but distinctively parsley in flavour. Rarely found in the UK, it is quite popular in Scandinavia and in central and eastern Europe. It is a cultivar of the more common leaf parsley and looks like a parsnip, although slightly whiter in appearance. Add it to soups and stews, or mash it with potatoes (see recipe, page 213) as a wonderful accompaniment to stews or game. The leaves are also edible. Hamburg parsley is harvested in the autumn and winter. In German, it's called *petersilienwurzel* or *wurzelpetersilie*.

Preparing parsley root

Scrub the root clean then remove the top and tail and peel (or don't – the peel has a lot of flavour, so in a stew or if roasting, you can leave it on). The root is used much like celeriac: cut into a julienne and eaten raw or quickly blanched; or in chunks, roasted, boiled or added to soups and stews.

KOHLRABI

We adore kohlrabi, and if you've never tried it, we urge you to give it ago. Picked fresh and tender, it can be peeled and eaten raw, with a crunchy, sweetish flavour almost like apple. It's fantastic sliced raw in salads, or lightly cooked.

People have been extolling its virtues in the UK for hundreds of years, and urging its wider adoption as a vegetable crop and animal feed. In the 1850s, one Mr W. Bennett of Cambridge addressed the Central Farmers' Club on the subject.

> He had been growing it, he said, for five years increasingly, and his opinion was that it was the most profitable crop upon the land, with the exception, perhaps, of mangold-wurzel. ... There was not much certainty about a crop of turnips after tares [deduction for wastage]. Once in five or six years they might succeed pretty well, but, generally speaking, they did not; whereas kohlrabi succeeded beyond a doubt. Being a hardy plant, it was difficult to kill, and for ewes and lambs it was as fine a food as they could have in March and April. His hoggets were now doing well on that grown on the fallows. He would strongly recommend, therefore, that where the land was good for anything, kohlrabi should be substituted for Swedes.

> Quoted in John Wilson, *Our Farm Crops* (1859)

No doubt the ewes, lambs and hoggets enjoyed the spring kohlrabi immensely – and so would the village folk have. It's a pity that some 150 years later, it is still hardly grown and continues to be a niche vegetable in the UK. (And just in passing, we do wish that hoggets – lambs that have been kept through the winter into their second year – were still widely available. They have an appealing muttony richness that has been lost to the English palate, not to speak of mutton itself. Check out the Mutton Renaissance Campaign for more on this.)

Preparing kohlrabi

Peel the kohlrabi and remove any tough fibrous parts that may be present in larger specimens, or ones that have been stressed during growing. You can then slice the tender flesh, or cut into julienne strips. The leaves of the immature plant can also be eaten. When raw, they have an appealing peppery flavour, or can be cooked like spinach.

Kohlrabi is the same species as wild cabbage, *Brassica oleracea*, as are many common vegetables, including broccoli, cauliflower, kale and Brussels sprouts, and cabbage itself. It is a cultivar group selected for its enlarged, almost spherical, mid-stem, which forms just above ground level. Preferring cool weather, it can be grown in the spring and autumn, and in frost-free winters. Most varieties are tenderest when small (about 5 to 10 centimetres across), and become tougher and less flavourful as they grow bigger. Some commercial cultivars have been developed that are still tender at larger sizes. Kohlrabi usually grows smaller in the spring, and a bit larger in the autumn.

Nettles and other foraged veg

> Nettles are so well known that they need no description; they may be found, by feeling, in the darkest night.

Culpeper's *Herbal*

It's hard to dispute Culpeper's point. Nevertheless, we feel that daytime nettle-gathering is preferable. That way, in addition to not getting stung, you can select young, light green nettle leaves – spring is the best time – far from roads and other sources of contamination. They are ubiquitous, free, and genuinely very tasty when wilted and buttered as you would spinach, or puréed into a silky soup.

This is not a book about foraging, but we wanted to briefly mention nettles and other wild greens, and mushrooms – two categories of overlooked and undercooked ingredients which fit well into this chapter.

In Greece we have been struck by the number of people who, having decided to put some greens on the table at lunchtime, head not to the supermarket but the hillside. Typically, they return with all manner of different leaves, some of which they will boil, others of which they serve in salads. In a relatively urban area of Switzerland a year or so back, one of us was told that the presence in the market of young people with wooden crates bursting with spiky green leaves signalled the beginning of the dandelion season. The hotel in which we were staying had procured some, and served them that night in a delicious bitter salad with lardons of bacon, cubes of Gruyère, croutons and a poached egg. This sort of spontaneous reflection of seasonality is very rarely found in UK hotels (let alone in budget establishments across the road from the railway station like this one) but that is hardly surprising given the fact that the knowledge required to pick wild greens – which appears to exist in most countries of continental Europe – does not seem to be engrained in our food culture at all (the taste for bitter greens certainly is; just witness the popularity of rocket and watercress). In the UK, picking wild greens on a hillside is seen more as an extreme sport than the restful, appetite stimulating, indeed life-reaffirming pre-prandial activity it actually is. There are simply hundreds of delicious, totally free wild greens out there if you know what you're looking for: alexanders, chicory, dandelion, dock, burdock, miner's lettuce and purslane, to name just a few. We'd encourage you to buy a book and learn about these matters. (Or search online for guided walks, led by people who really know what they're doing.) Having learned, teach your children.

Then there are wild fungi, numerous species of which are edible. Of course, you have to be careful. It's true that there are some species of mushroom which – even in tiny quantities – are deadly poisonous. But there are not many, and you can forage for mushrooms perfectly safely if you use your head. Our own tip, which might seem counter-intuitive, is that the worst thing you can do when contemplating going out mushrooming for the first time is to buy yourself a huge book which identifies every fungi variety known to humankind. You will get totally and utterly lost trying to identify your harvest (some of which, when you get home, might be poisonous anyway – and will probably therefore have tainted all the others). We approach things from precisely the opposite direction: we're interested in gastronomy, not mycology. So, learn to identify one or two species with absolute certainty, either from a book or, better still, from someone who really knows what they're doing – the field mushroom, penny bun boletus (or cép or porcini), the bay bolete and the chanterelle, for example. You simply cannot make mistakes with these.

We learned this technique by accident, since one of us was introduced to mushroom picking by an Italian chef who wasn't interested in anything except his beloved porcini. Having crawled under the fence bordering a famous golf course in the Home Counties of the UK at half-past three in the morning, and diving for cover at the slightest noise more in the manner of commandos than mushroom pickers, we began to notice fungi everywhere. But if they weren't porcini, Giuseppe (whom a close mushrooming friend later christened 'Joe Cep') simply wasn't interested: we never found out what these other fungi were and didn't bother picking them. Sure, we probably missed a whole bunch of other species that are edible, but there are few mushrooms as unforgettably edible as fresh porcini.

And how unforgettable the experience can be. Arise at dawn and take a small camping stove into the woods with you too, a battered old steel pan or wok, a clove of garlic, a knob of butter in a piece of foil, a couple of bread rolls and a flask of red wine. Once you have your baskets full, find a quiet spot – it will be between six and seven o'clock in the morning by now – and cook up your fresh porcini with garlic and butter. Enjoy them with your bread rolls, wine and birdsong.

You will approach the rest of the day differently to other days. You may find your life subtly changed. That is what real good food can do.

Misshapen vegetables

While we're on the subject of ugly vegetables, it is important to mention another type of overlooked ingredient: that of cosmetically 'flawed' but perfectly tasty and nutritious vegetables and fruit that are dumped in massive quantities by growers and retailers. This is a huge problem: about one-third of produce is discarded before it reaches our shops, much of it for spurious cosmetic reasons – too big, too small, too lumpy, too ugly. In the UK alone, this amounts to hundreds of thousands of tons of perfectly good food being ploughed back into fields or sent to landfill every year. It's not just a waste of food; it's a waste of the scarce resources – land, water, energy – that are needed to produce it.

There has thankfully been growing public awareness of this needless waste. In 2008 and 2009, the European Union eased its strict marketing classifications on a range of fruit and vegetables, making it easier for shops to sell different sized and shaped produce. This was the end of much-ridiculed requirements that 'Class I' bananas be 'free of abnormal curvature' and at least 14 centimetres in length, or that cucumbers must be 'practically straight' with a curvature of no more than 10 millimetres for each 10 centimetres in length.

More recently, campaigners such as Tristram Stuart and celebrity chefs such as Hugh Fearnley-Whittingstall have taken the battle to the supermarkets, who maintain needlessly strict purchasing standards. This has resulted in Sainsbury's, Asda and other major retailers taking a number of important steps, including selling misshapen produce at a discount with branding such as 'wonky veg' or 'beautiful on the inside'. There is a risk, though, that such moves reinforce the idea that naturally grown produce should be judged by cosmetic criteria and conform to some Platonic ideal, when we should be building understanding among consumers that vegetables grow in fields and that a bit of mud, discolouration or knobbliness is normal. We support calls by campaigners for supermarkets to go further than just selling 'ugly' produce at a discount; they need to relax their cosmetic standards so that a wider range of shapes and sizes can be found in their flagship produce sections. Some retailers are starting to move in this direction, but they need to go much further.

We'd be more sympathetic if supermarkets were pursuing a Platonic ideal of quality and flavour – rejecting tomatoes that weren't delectable enough, or fruit that was picked too early, forced to inhale ethylene gas, and just didn't taste any good. But the fact is, it's precisely the opposite. There's often a negative correlation between looks and taste: the pursuit of blemish-free geometric perfection distracts from or is even inimical to the pursuit of flavour. Growers, under pressure from supermarket purchasing specifications, have moved away from tasty varieties to ones that have a more regular appearance or a longer shelf life. Consider those 'heirloom' varieties at farmer's markets that are often weird looking or misshapen but taste great. (Although we suspect that sometimes the pendulum swings too far in the other direction, and now that retailers have jumped on the bandwagon, odd-looking varieties are sold at a high price because of an heirloom label, rather than because they necessarily taste amazing.)

Tackling the problem of discarded produce is very much linked to the central theme of this book. There is a global food crisis. Agriculture is already the biggest contributor to global warming, the largest user of our limited supplies of fresh water (and one of the biggest polluters of it), and the major cause of wildlife extinction. And it is estimated that total food production will need to double over the next 30 to 40 years to meet the needs of a growing and more prosperous global population.

Part of the solution is to reduce food waste. Another – the theme of this book – is to shift our eating habits to increase our consumption of more sustainable ingredients or under-utilised cuts of meat and fish. Why convert thousands of acres of forest or other wild land to farming when there are millions of rabbits and squirrels and octopus and ugly fish and discarded cheeks and feet that are perfectly edible – and more than that, are delicious and healthy? Reducing food waste and changing what we eat both require altering our purchasing habits, but more fundamentally they require a shift in our relationship with food. We must re-embrace meat and fish and vegetables as natural products – things that come with blood or mud and in different shapes and sizes, things that taste of something – not as processed products that are as disposable and tasteless as the plastic packaging they come wrapped in. Eat more ugly food!

RECIPES

All recipes serve 4 unless otherwise noted.

Wine Braised Root Vegetables

A most excellent stew made from, well, whatever you have to hand – plus some wine.

1kg assorted root vegetables, cut into 2 cm chunks (aim for a balance of flavours/textures)

100g shallots, thinly sliced

3 sprigs thyme, leaves chopped

30g butter (plus a little more to finish)

200ml white wine (say, a good chardonnay)

200ml chicken stock (preferably homemade)

1 sprig of flat-leaf parsley, leaves chopped

salt, freshly-ground black pepper and white wine vinegar

1. Sauté the shallots and thyme in 20g of the butter until softened (2–3 minutes). Add the wine, bring to the boil, flame off the alcohol, then simmer until reduced by half.

2. Add the vegetables, stock and a little salt, and simmer very gently, covered, until the vegetables are tender – about 10–20 minutes, depending on the vegetables. Remove the vegetables from the liquid and keep warm.

3. Meanwhile, boil the braising liquid to reduce to a thick sauce. Whisk in the remaining butter and season to taste with salt and pepper, as well as a little vinegar. Pour over the vegetables and serve, garnished with the parsley.

You can make a hearty, warming winter version of this dish with red wine. You might like to add 200g sliced mushrooms, sautéed after the shallots until most of their liquid has evaporated before adding the wine. If you go this route, consider a few dried porcini for depth as well (soaked, chopped and added to the wine reduction with their soaking liquid, strained to remove any grit). Some rosemary might be nice, and you might substitute red wine vinegar at the end.

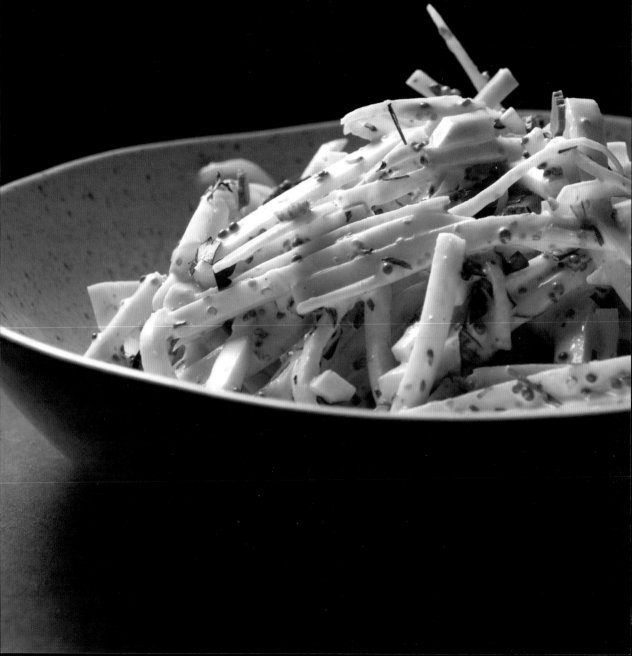

Roast Mangel-Wurzel

Roasting mangel-wurzels whole keeps their golden colour (depending on the cultivar), and intensifies the flavour.

500g mangel-wurzel

olive oil

1 sprig rosemary

salt and freshly-ground black pepper

butter

1 sprig flat-leaf parsley

1. Pre-heat the oven to 180°C.

2. Remove the leaves of the mangel-wurzel so that about 1 cm of stalks remain attached to the root. Trim the tail if it is long. Wash carefully, scrubbing with a vegetable brush to remove all the dirt, then dry.

3. Lay on a sheet of aluminium foil and brush with olive oil all over. Add the rosemary and a generous amount of salt and freshly-ground pepper. Place a second sheet of aluminium foil on top, and roll up the sides to form a tightly-wrapped parcel. If using more than one mangel-wurzel, wrap each one separately.

4. Place the foil parcel(s) into the oven and roast for 40–60 minutes, until tender. (To check, pierce with a paring knife; it should go in easily, but will have slightly more resistance than a cooked potato.)

5. Remove from the oven and when cool enough to handle, trim the tops and bottoms and rub off the skins with paper towel. Cut into chunks, season well and serve with a knob of softened butter and chopped parsley.

We have yet to encounter an ugly root vegetable that does not respond well to this technique. Try it with beetroot, Jerusalem artichoke, celeriac, parsley root or kohlrabi, adjusting the cooking time depending on the size of the vegetable – 30 minutes works for Jerusalem artichokes, and you may need over 2 hours for a decent-sized celeriac. Try thyme, bay leaf or oregano instead of the rosemary, and you could add some roughly chopped garlic to the foil package as well.

Mangel-Wurzel Confit

A fabulous side dish that's perfect served with squirrel, duck breast or game.

200g mangel-wurzel slices, 3-4 mm thick (without peel)
20g butter
10g sugar

1. Cook the mangel-wurzel slices in boiling salted water for 4 minutes. Remove and refresh in ice water. Drain.

2. In a sauté pan, melt the butter and add the sugar, along with 30ml water. Stir until the sugar has dissolved. Add the mangel-wurzel and simmer, turning occasionally until the liquid just starts to caramelise and the mangel-wurzel is tender but still firm. (Add a little more water if necessary.) Serve immediately.

Wilted Mangel-Wurzel Tops

The leaves and stems of mangel-wurzels are very much like Swiss chard, and rather more delicate. They make a perfect complement to rabbit confit (page 158). Swiss chard can be substituted for the mangel-wurzel tops.

400g mangel-wurzel leaves with stems
10g shallots, finely chopped
1 sprig thyme, leaves chopped
2 cloves garlic, finely chopped
10ml olive oil (or fat from rabbit confit)
220ml chicken stock (preferably homemade)
40g Dijon mustard
60g crème fraiche
5g chives, finely chopped
sea salt

1. Get the mangel-wurzel leaves ready. Wash well, then separate the stem and hard central vein from the leaf. Cut the leaves into 5 cm-wide strips and the stems into 5 cm-long pieces.

2. Briefly sauté the shallots, thyme and garlic in the oil to soften. Add the chicken stock and simmer for 4–5 minutes to reduce a little. Stir in the

mustard and crème fraiche. Add salt to taste (if serving with confit, go light on the salt).

3. Meanwhile, cook the mangel-wurzel leaves. Put half a centimetre of water into a saucepan large enough to hold the leaves, add the stems, cover, then bring to the boil and simmer for 2 minutes until just tender. Add the leaves (there should be a little water remaining in the pan), cover, and cook until wilted, about another 2 minutes.

4. Add the cooked leaves and stems to the sauce, leaving behind any water. Stir so that the leaves are separated and well-coated. Remove from the heat and stir in the chives.

Mangel-Wurzel Beer

Never having made this ourselves, we defer to the authority of Mrs Dalgairns, author of *The Practice of Cookery, Adapted to the Business of Every Day Life* (1829), who assures the reader that 'by this receipt, good keeping table-beer will be obtained'. We reproduce it as originally published.

> For a ten-gallon cask, boil in fourteen gallons of water sixty pounds of mangel-wurzel, which has been well washed and sliced across, putting some kind of weight on the roots to keep them under water; having boiled an hour and a half, they may be taken out, well broken, and all the liquor pressed from the roots; put it, and that in which they were boiled, on again to boil, with four ounces of hops; let them boil about an hour and a half, then cool the liquor, as quickly as possible, to 70° Fahrenheit; strain it through a thick cloth laid over a sieve or drainer; put it into the vat with about six ounces of good yeast, stir it well, cover it, and let it stand twenty-four hours; if the yeast has then well risen, skim it off, and barrel the beer, keeping back the thick sediment. While the fermentation goes on in the cask, it may be filled up with the beer left over, or any other kind at hand; when the fermentation ceases, which may be in two or three days, the cask must be bunged up, and in a few days more, the beer may be used from the cask, or bottled.

> These small proportions are here given to suit the convenience of the humblest labourer; but the beer will be better made in larger quantities; and its strength may be increased by adding a greater proportion of mangel-wurzel.

Jerusalem Artichoke Soup

We love Jerusalem artichoke soup, with its rich earthy and nutty taste. But don't just take our word for it: in 2002 the French city of Nice reportedly voted it 'best vegetable for soup'; we have no confirmation of this, but the Internet says so. Canadian Prime Minister Justin Trudeau also revealed in December

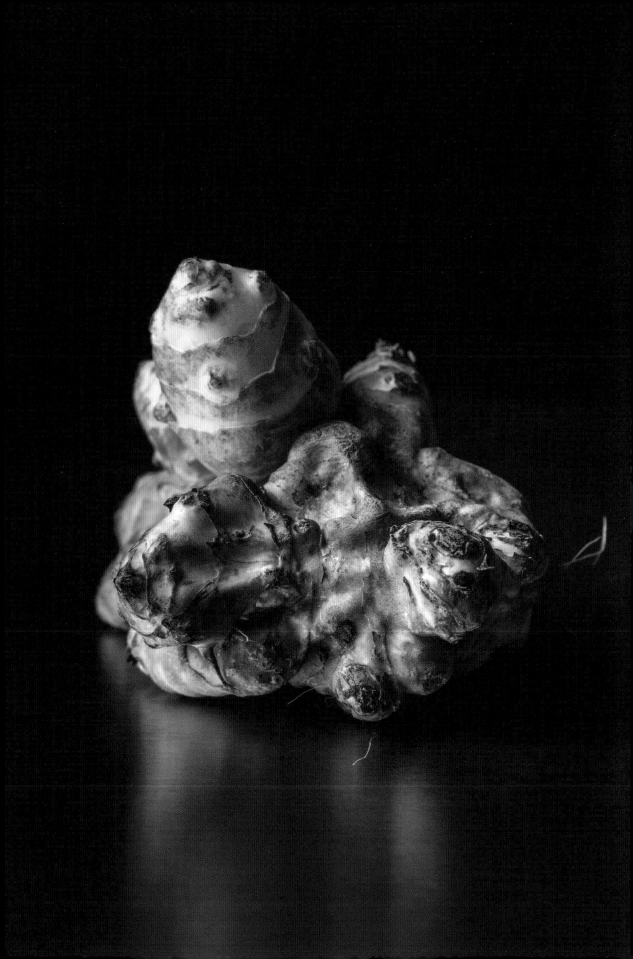

2015 that his favourite French word is *topinambour*, which means 'Jerusalem artichoke'. We like to think that, like us, he's a fan of the soup rather than just the sound of the word, but he didn't elaborate.

400g Jerusalem artichokes, washed but not peeled, cut into 2 cm chunks
10ml olive oil
40g bacon or pancetta, diced
1 clove garlic, chopped
180g leek, white and light green parts only, thinly sliced
80g celery, thinly sliced
80g floury potato, cut into 2 cm chunks
750ml chicken stock (homemade)
10g salt
bouquet garni
(8 peppercorns, bay leaf and 3 sprigs thyme, tied in muslin or leek leaves)
40ml thick cream
freshly-ground white pepper

1. Heat the oil in a large saucepan, and brown the bacon well. Remove the bacon pieces and reserve.

2. Add the garlic, leek and celery to the pan and sauté in the bacon fat until very soft, but not browned.

3. Add the Jerusalem artichokes (reserving a little for garnish) and potato and cook over very low heat, with the lid on, for 15 minutes. Turn up the heat, add the stock, salt and bouquet garni and simmer, uncovered, until the Jerusalem artichokes and potato are soft, about 30 minutes.

4. Remove the bouquet garni, then purée the soup and pass through a fine-mesh sieve into a clean pan.

5. Place the pan over low heat. Stir in the cream, bring to a gentle simmer, and add a few turns of white pepper and more salt as needed.

6. Serve, garnished with the bacon pieces and some raw Jerusalem artichoke, peeled and grated.

Our top tip for Jerusalem artichokes: Don't peel them. The skins are edible, and contain a lot of the characteristic earthy flavour.

This soup is delicious with poached scallops. That may sound unusual, but it really is a marriage made in heaven, courtesy of Margaret Costa's excellent *Four Seasons Cookery Book*. If you are going to use scallops, we'd recommend omitting the bacon from the recipe. Just lightly poach a few scallops in a little milk, cut them into a dice and add to the finished soup, along with the warm poaching milk, then serve.

Jerusalem Artichokes with Cream

Simple, but delightful.

1kg Jerusalem artichokes, peeled and cut into thin (3–4 mm) slices
80g butter
salt and freshly-ground black pepper
100ml double cream
2 sprigs flat-leaf parsley, leaves chopped
freshly-grated nutmeg
lemon juice

1. Melt the butter in a large sauté pan, add the Jerusalem artichoke slices, and turn to coat in the butter. Season with salt and pepper, then add just enough water to cover.

2. Simmer without a lid until the water has nearly evaporated and the Jerusalem artichokes are tender. Stir in the cream and most of the the parsley and simmer for a minute or two.

3. Remove from the heat and stir in a little grated nutmeg, and a few drops of lemon juice and adjust the seasoning. Serve, garnished with a little more chopped parsley.

Roast Jerusalem Artichoke, Goat's Cheese and Hazelnut Salad

This is adapted from Hugh Fearnley-Whittingstall, who says 'the earthy flavour of the roasted artichokes is delicious with toasted hazelnuts'. We agree. Keeping the skins on adds flavour, and prevents the artichokes breaking up too much when you toss them into the salad.

650g Jerusalem artichokes, washed well but not peeled
60ml extra-virgin olive oil
5g salt

1-2 bay leaves

5ml hazelnut oil

half a lemon

80g whole hazelnuts, toasted and de-skinned

80g hard goat's cheese, cut into small chunks

rocket leaves (a couple of handfuls)

salt and freshly-ground black pepper

1. Put a large roasting pan in the oven and pre-heat to 180°C.

2. Cut the Jerusalem artichokes into even-sized chunks (roughly, quarters). Coat with 40ml of the olive oil, the salt and bay leaf.

3. Put into the hot pan and roast until lightly golden, about 35 minutes, turning them about half-way through. When cooked, remove the pan from the oven and set aside to cool slightly.

4. Meanwhile, whisk together the remaining 20ml of olive oil with the hazelnut oil, drizzle over the warm artichokes, squeeze some lemon juice over them and season with salt and a few turns of black pepper. Mix gently with your hands to combine well, then add the nuts, goat's cheese and rocket. Serve.

Salsify with Tarragon

Salsify pairs fantastically with a creamy sauce – the classic French preparations, given by Escoffier, are salsifis à la crème and salsifis au gratin. Both are excellent. But we particularly love this recipe, adapted from Sophie Grigson.

600g salsify

15g butter

30ml dry vermouth

60g crème fraiche

1 sprig tarragon, leaves chopped

salt

1. Either boil or braise according to one of the basic methods described below.

2. Heat the butter in a sauté pan until foaming. Add the salsify and turn until just starting to colour (2–3 minutes), then add the vermouth. Continue to cook, turning the salsify, until nearly all the vermouth has evaporated.

3. Add the crème fraiche, tarragon and some salt and simmer until the sauce has thickened a little and is starting to coat the salsify. Adjust seasoning and serve.

Basic techniques for cooking salsify

Here are two basic cooking techniques for preparing salsify. Either is perfect as a side-dish.

Basic method for boiling:

Wash the salsify and remove the skin by scraping or peeling. Cut into 3 inch lengths, slicing the thicker parts into two or four lengthways so they are all about the same thickness. Keep the pieces in acidulated water (7ml vinegar per litre) until ready to use. Cook in a large pot of salted and acidulated water at a rolling boil. Start checking doneness after 15–20 minutes, and cook until tender but still slightly firm. Remove and drain on paper towels. (If you are not going to use them immediately, shock them in ice water before draining, to halt the cooking process.)

Basic method for braising:

Clean and cut the salsify as for boiling (above). Place in a saucepan large enough to take them in a single layer (at most a double layer) and add olive oil to just cover. Put the lid on the saucepan and place over low heat to braise very gently, without colouring, until tender. Shake the pan occasionally. Start checking doneness after 20 minutes; but be aware that the cooking time can vary considerably. Remove and drain on paper towels.

This method of braising gently in olive oil (or any other fat of your choice) also works fabulously for other vegetables, such as asparagus and carrots. Many of their flavour and colour molecules are soluble in water but not in oil. Boiling therefore removes flavour and colour that braising in oil does not. The difference in taste and appearance can be striking.

To finish:

After cooking by either boiling or braising, finish by heating some butter in a sauté pan until foaming. Add the salsify and turn until just starting to colour. Serve with chopped parsley and a squeeze of lemon.

Beef and Burdock Rolls

Known in Japanese as *Yawata-maki*, after the city of Yawata (near Kyoto) which was famous for its abundant burdock plants, this is a glorious combination of crunchy burdock and succulent beef. The dish is sometimes also made with eel fillet instead of beef.

4 burdock roots

700g highly-marbled Wagyu beef (pre-cut into sukiyaki slices if available)

For the marinade:

400ml dashi (from instant granules)

40ml mirin

30ml light soy sauce

For basting:

45ml sake

90ml mirin

90ml dark soy sauce

Japanese pepper (*sancho*), ground

a few young burdock leaves for garnish (optional)

1. Gently scrub the burdock roots and remove any rootlets. Do not peel. Cut into 10cm-long julienne strips of even thickness, keeping cut strips in cold water to prevent discolouration.

2. Boil the strips until softened (about 5 minutes, depending on thickness) in plenty of boiling water which has been acidulated with 7ml of vinegar per litre. This will prevent discolouration. Once soft, remove the strips and refresh in ice water.

3. Combine the marinade ingredients, add the burdock strips, and leave for 3-4 hours. Remove and drain on paper towels.

4. The beef should be cut into very thin slices, as for *sukiyaki*. You can buy this pre-sliced, or ask your butcher to do it for you. To do it yourself, half-freeze the block of beef to make it firmer and easier to cut. Arrange some beef slices, slightly overlapping, into a continuous sheet about 10 cm wide (the same width as the burdock strips) and a similar length. Lay about 10 burdock strips across the sheet of beef, and roll them up tightly in the beef. Secure with butcher's string if necessary. Repeat until you have used all the burdock and the beef.

Japanese ingredients

Most of these ingredients are easily available in Japanese groceries, or even many Western supermarkets, including mirin (a rice wine for cooking), sake and Japanese pepper (sold pre-ground in little shakers). Dashi is a wonderful Japanese stock, made from *konbu* kelp and dried bonito flakes. As with other stocks, normally we would recommend making your own, which gives an unparalleled subtlety and depth of flavour. For the purpose of the marinade in this dish, however, it is fine to use instant dashi that you can buy in packets from Japanese shops.

5. Combine the basting ingredients, place the beef rolls into a baking pan, and pour over the basting mixture. Marinate for one hour, turning the rolls occasionally. Remove the rolls and reserve the basting mixture.

6. To finish, secure the rolls with dampened bamboo skewers and grill over charcoal until the meat is cooked medium. Baste with the reserved mixture while grilling. Alternatively, sauté the rolls in a pan with a little oil until lightly browned, then continue cooking in a little of the basting liquid. Serve, dusted with Japanese pepper and some pickles on the side, and some young raw burdock leaves if you have some.

Burdock Kinpira Style

Kinpira is a Japanese technique for sautéing and simmering root vegetables in soy sauce and mirin, commonly used to prepare burdock as a side dish. The technique works well with other root vegetables including carrot, mangel-wurzel and celery root.

1 burdock root

neutral oil

30ml sake

30ml dark soy sauce

10g sugar

Japanese red pepper flakes (*ichimi*)

1. Gently scrub the burdock roots and remove any rootlets. Do not peel. Cut into thin shavings, as if you were sharpening a pencil with a penknife. Keep the shavings in cold water to prevent discolouration.

2. Heat a little oil in sauté pan, and stir-fry over high heat until the burdock has softened a little, about 3 minutes. Add the sake, soy sauce and sugar to the pan and continue sautéing until the liquid has almost completely evaporated. Add Japanese red pepper flakes to taste.

Celeriac Remoulade

This classic recipe brings out perfectly the wonderful celery flavour. It also works really well with kohlrabi, or a mixture of kohlrabi and apple.

300g celeriac

35g wholegrain mustard

5g capers, finely chopped
25g cornichons, finely chopped
juice of 1 lemon
1 sprig flat-leaf parsley, leaves chopped
4 sprigs tarragon, leaves chopped
150g mayonnaise
salt and freshly-ground black pepper

1. Peel the celeriac and cut into fine strips. Toss with the mustard, capers, cornichons and lemon juice.

2. Add the herbs to the mixture, stir in the mayonnaise and season with salt and freshly-ground pepper.

Salad of Celeriac, Radish and Pomegranate

A wonderful combination of flavours and textures, adapted from a recipe by Jacob Kennedy.

60g chunk of peeled celeriac
8 radishes, washed
60g Pecorino Romano cheese
40g pomegranate seeds
2 sprigs flat-leaf parsley, leaves picked

For the dressing:

90ml extra virgin olive oil
15ml white balsamic vinegar
10ml lemon juice
salt and freshly-ground black pepper

1. Whisk together the dressing ingredients and adjust seasoning.

2. Cut the radishes into wafer-thin slices using a mandolin. Shave the celeriac and cheese using a vegetable peeler.

3. Combine all the ingredients together with enough of the dressing to coat lightly, and serve.

Celeriac Soup

300g celeriac

200g floury potatoes

250ml milk

50ml double cream

salt and freshly-ground black pepper

butter or crème fraiche

1 sprig flat-leaf parsley (or tender leaves from stem celery), leaves chopped

1. Peel the celeriac and potato and cut into equal-sized chunks. Add the milk, season with salt and pepper, and simmer until the potato and celeriac are soft.

2. Purée the soup and pass through a sieve into a clean pan.

3. Place the pan over a low heat. Stir in the cream, bring to a gentle simmer, and add more salt and pepper as needed. Serve, garnished with a small knob of butter or spoon of crème fraiche, and chopped parsley or celery leaves.

Celeriac Gratin

This dish really amplifies the celeriac flavour. Eat as a main dish, or as a really great accompaniment to rabbit (halve the quantities to serve 4 as a side dish). For the best results, use an aged Gruyère which has a stronger, nuttier flavour (labelled 'vieux' or 'réserve').

1kg celeriac

500g floury potatoes

120ml thick cream

60g butter

pinch of saffron threads

1 clove garlic, finely chopped

180g Gruyère cheese (preferably aged), coarsely grated

salt and white pepper

1 sprig flat-leaf parsley, leaves chopped

1. Pre-heat the oven to 200°C.

2. Peel the celeriac and potato and cut into equal-sized chunks. Place into separate pans with enough salted water to cover. Bring to the boil and simmer until soft. Strain and reserve the celeriac and potatoes separately.

3. In a small pan, bring the cream to a boil and add the butter, saffron and garlic. Reduce the heat and simmer for 5 minutes.

4. Purée the celeriac in a food processor, gradually incorporating the cream mixture. Coarsely mash the potatoes, then fold in the celeriac purée, 120g of the grated Gruyère and a generous seasoning of salt and freshly-ground white pepper.

5. Butter a 20 cm x 20 cm (or equivalent) baking dish. For individual servings, use 4 ramekins of 300ml capacity. Spoon the mixture into the dish or ramekins and sprinkle with the parsley and remaining Gruyère.

6. Bake for 15 minutes, or until the mixture is heated through and a golden-brown crust has formed.

Both kohlrabi and salsify work well cooked this way.

Hamburg Parsley Mash

Boiled potatoes just cry out for butter and parsley. This mash with parsley root goes one better – it's perfect with chicken casseroles, meaty stews and game dishes.

200g Hamburg parsley root, trimmed, peeled and cut into 1cm slices
500g floury potatoes, peeled and cut into 1 cm slices
80g butter, cut into small cubes
a little hot milk or cream
salt and freshly-ground white pepper

1. Rinse the potato slices in cold water to remove any starch. Boil the parsley root and potatoes in salted water until very tender. Drain in a colander and leave for a few minutes until the moisture has evaporated.

2. Return to the warm pan and mash with a potato masher or ricer, then stir in the butter until fully incorporated.

3. Gradually add the hot milk until the desired consistency has been achieved. Season with salt and white pepper to taste. Serve warm.

Hamburg Parsley Soup with Chestnuts

Earthy, silky, parsley-ey. With crunchy, nutty chestnuts. What's not to like?

700g Hamburg parsley root, trimmed, scrubbed (not peeled)
and cut into 1 cm slices
30g butter
100g onion, thinly sliced
1 clove garlic, finely chopped
850ml chicken stock (preferably homemade)
bouquet garni (8 peppercorns, bay leaf and 3 sprigs thyme, tied in muslin or
leek leaves)
50ml double cream
4 whole roasted chestnuts, peeled and shaved very thinly
salt and freshly-ground white pepper

1. Heat the butter in a large saucepan, and sauté the onion until very soft, but not browned. Add the garlic and cook for another 1-2 minutes.

2. Add the parsley root (reserving a little for the garnish) and cook over low heat, with the lid on, until it has softened a little, about 10 minutes. Turn up the heat, add the stock, the bouquet garni and some salt and simmer, uncovered, until the parsley root is very soft, about 30 minutes.

3. Remove the bouquet garni, then purée the soup and pass through a fine-mesh sieve into a clean pan.

4. Place the pan over low heat. Stir in the cream, bring to a gentle simmer, and add a few turns of white pepper and more salt as needed.

5. Serve, garnished with the chestnut slices and some raw parsley root, peeled and grated.

You can also try adding parsley root to any of the celeriac recipes above – we suggest replacing one-third of the celeriac, to get a mixture of the two flavours.

Chicken with Parsley Root and Chanterelles

Parsley root goes perfectly with chicken. Chicken goes perfectly with chanterelles.

4 chicken breasts (skin on)
butter

250g parsley root, trimmed and peeled (reserve leaves for garnish)
200ml chicken stock (preferably homemade)
lemon juice
100g chanterelles
50g hazelnuts, whole with skins removed
hazelnut oil
salt and freshly-ground black pepper

1. Pre-heat oven to 200°C.

2. Rub the chicken breasts with butter, season with salt and pepper and wrap each in aluminium foil. Place in a tray and cook to an internal temperature of 65°C, about 20 minutes (flip the foil packets over after 10 minutes for even cooking).

3. Meanwhile, cut the parsley root lengthways into four. Place in a pan, cover with chicken stock and add some salt and a good squeeze of lemon juice. Simmer, covered, until tender. Remove and reserve.

4. In a hot pan, sauté the mushrooms in butter with a little salt until most of the moisture has evaporated. Add the hazelnuts and sauté for a little longer. Remove and reserve.

5. Brown the chicken breasts in butter, skin side down, until golden. In a separate pan, brown the parsley root in hazelnut oil briefly over high heat.

6. Slice the chicken breast and serve with the mushrooms and parsley root, garnished with some leaves from the parsley root (or flat-leaf parsley).

This dish goes well with wilted mangel-wurzel tops or Swiss chard (recipe, page 202), which provides a sauce. Alternatively, you could reduce the chicken stock in which the parsley roots were simmered, whisk in some crème fraiche and Dijon mustard, and season with salt and pepper.

Salad of Kohlrabi and Fennel

An endearingly crisp and crunchy concoction.

150g peeled kohlrabi
150g trimmed fennel bulb
30g rocket leaves
30g hazelnuts, toasted

For the dressing:
90ml extra virgin olive oil
30ml lemon juice
salt and freshly-ground white pepper

1. Whisk together the dressing ingredients and adjust seasoning.

2. Remove the core from the fennel, then cut into wafer-thin slices using a mandolin. Slice the peeled kohlrabi thinly or shave using a vegetable peeler.

3. Combine all the ingredients together with enough of the dressing to coat lightly, and serve.

Butter-Braised Kohlrabi

Excellent as an accompaniment to hearty meat dishes, such as *daube* (page 66), rabbit or squirrel.

800g peeled kohlrabi
40g unsalted butter
10g finely chopped shallot
5g caster sugar
5ml white wine vinegar
100ml chicken stock or vegetable stock (preferably homemade)
salt and freshly-ground black pepper

1. Cut the kohlrabi into slices about 1 cm thick, then crossways into 1cm wide batons.

2. Melt the butter in a sauté pan over medium heat, add the shallot and cook until soft, about 2–3 minutes, stirring often.

3. Add the kohlrabi, sugar, vinegar and about 60ml of stock. Season with salt and plenty of pepper.

4. Bring to a simmer, cover the pan and cook gently until the kohlrabi has softened a little, about 5–10 minutes, adding a little more stock if necessary.

5. Uncover the pan and cook for a few minutes more, swirling the pan regularly, until the sauce has reduced to glaze that covers the kohlrabi, which should now be tender. Before serving, taste for seasoning and add more salt, pepper and a few drops of vinegar as needed.

Nettle Soup

A verdant, luxurious soup. Nettles should be picked in spring when they are most tender; go for the young tops, without the fibrous stems – and don't forget protective gloves. Nettle tea is suggested by herbalists as a mild laxative, but we've never noticed any particular impact from a bowl of soup.

400g young nettle tops (a grocery-bag full, rinsed only if they need it)
15ml olive oil
200g onion, sliced
300g leeks, sliced
300g floury potatoes, peeled and cut into 1 cm slices
1 litre chicken stock (homemade makes all the difference here)
80g double cream
salt and freshly-ground black pepper

1. Sauté the onions and leeks in the olive oil until very soft, but not browned. Add the potatoes and the chicken stock and simmer until the potatoes are starting to fall apart.

2. Add the nettles and cook briefly until wilted, about one minute.

3. Purée the soup, and pass through a fine-mesh sieve into a clean pan.

4. Place the pan over low heat, stir in the cream, return to a simmer and add salt and pepper to taste.

5. Serve, perhaps garnished with a young dead-nettle leaf – which looks and tastes the part, but won't sting your guests.

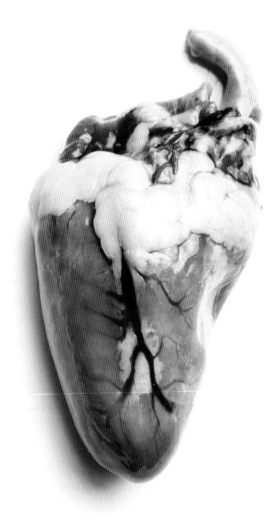

7. GIBLETS

Talk of strange relics led to mention of the heart of a French king preserved at Nuneham in a silver casket. Dr Buckland, whilst looking at it exclaimed, 'I have eaten many strange things, but have never eaten the heart of a king before,' and, before any one could hinder him, he had gobbled it up, and the precious relic was lost for ever.

Augustus Hare's description of the moment William Buckland, Dean of Westminster, ate the preserved heart of Louis XIV (from his *The Story of My Life*, Vol. V, 1900)

On eating everything

During their weekly shop the majority of British shoppers will purchase a package or two marked with a notice containing the word 'giblets'. Ironically enough, however, far from describing something that is contained within the package, such notices are a perfect reflection of the kind of problems with Anglo-Saxon food culture that we are keen to point out: 'Without giblets', they proclaim.

The trend towards mass-produced supermarket birds – anaemic, hormone-stuffed chickens and brine-injected, fake-butter-flavoured turkeys – has done more than just create foul fowl, it has taken away some of the best bits of the bird: the giblets, neck, and feet that once came with the just-slaughtered bird, and which, until recently, were stuffed into the cavity. Even quality, free-range birds now come less and less often with the accompanying little bag of bits. And that's a real pity, because giblets are fantastic (so are feet, as discussed in a previous chapter). The heart, gizzard and liver of birds are easy to turn into wonderful dishes – and we're not just talking stuffing or gravy (we say use the neck and wingtips for gravy, and we're very much against that big mass of undercooked giblet stuffing in an overcooked bird).

Precisely why birds no longer come with giblets, we don't know; moreover, we haven't been able to find out. It has been suggested that cases of salmonella poisoning in the 1980s in the UK and US, and the subsequent media frenzy, put paid to the practice. We're not sure. Even when giblets were included, most poultry processing plants dealt with the giblets separately (so the giblets you actually got with your bird were certainly never from the bird you had actually bought). We suspect their disappearance was primarily down to lack of demand, which may or may not have been exacerbated by salmonella scares and so on. Culinary demand for giblets is now so low in the UK that most of them are sold to pet-food manufacturers (though in the southern states of the US, hearts and gizzards in particular are much sought after for use in 'soul food' cooking).

Giblets are cheap, sustainable, and they're utterly delicious. When you buy a bird, make sure you get its giblets: buy everything, eat everything. By the end of this chapter we hope you will be a convert.

For the best part of twenty years there has been something of an offal revival underway in the Britain and the US. In the world of professional cookery, the 'nose-to-tail' approach championed by Fergus Henderson in the UK, and the championing of Henderson in the US by Anthony Bourdain, has not only altered our perception of what kind of dishes we might be served in restaurants or gastro-pubs (lamb shanks are quite common now, ox-cheeks becoming more so) but also resulted in the publication of a range of books. In addition to Henderson's own excellent books we might add *Odd Bits: How to Cook the Rest of the Animal* by Jennifer McLagan, a book that raises questions similar to the ones we address in our series. How is it that shoppers have become so far removed from the source of the shrink-wrapped fillets on sale in the supermarket? Why do so many people recoil from an ingredient just because of where it comes from? Why don't we eat the whole beast?

Our own favourite, albeit not a recent one, is a bold, uncompromising and inexplicably long out-of-print volume by Jana Allen and Margaret Gin (of *Maggie Gin* stir-fry sauces fame) entitled *Innards and Other Variety Meats*. Allen and Gin include a recipe that calls for a quart of lambs testicles. That takes a lot of balls.

We're 100 per cent behind this revival – indeed, we urge you to buy and read these books – but we do recognise that ox liver and pigs kidneys (or, for that matter, spleen, lung, brains and testicles) aren't to everyone's taste. Giblets, however, are a completely different story. Chicken hearts, which, contrary to popular belief, have neither a strong smell nor a remotely strong flavour, are delicious. Marinate them in garlic and lemon, then grill them over charcoal (or on a barred griddle pan) gaucho style (see recipe on page 238) and sprinkle generously with sea salt: these hearts are hard to beat. Prepared well, bird livers don't have the typical offal flavour we associate with pig liver or ox liver, just a delicate richness that soothes body and soul: think Pâté de Foie (see our recipe on page 245).

And beyond specific dishes such as these, we would also encourage you to think of giblets, particularly the heart and liver, as condiments, which can immeasurably improve a whole range of dishes. Added to a Ragù alla bolognese, they give a fantastic depth of flavour, which is particularly good for lasagne; or add to soup pot-au-feu for a richer broth; or freeze cubes of giblet stock to add to any dish where a meaty richness is called for (and ok, gravy too). Indeed, while beyond the scope of this chapter, a Daube de boeuf Bourguignon (recipe on page 66) made with half-and-half ox cheeks and chopped ox heart is a thing of wonder. We have even made it with just heart.

As for the embalmed heart of French royalty (see the epigraph to this chapter), we admit that is a long way beyond the line we draw between what we are prepared to eat and what we are not: eating everything does not entail eating anything. William Buckland was, however, an interesting man and, we feel, worthy of a passing mention. As well as being a distinguished geologist (he was Oxford's first reader in Geology), archaeologist and pioneering coprologist (coprology is the study of fossilised animal droppings), he was unofficial curator of the Ashmolean Museum in Oxford and, having been ordained in 1808, was later appointed Dean of Westminster. Buckland, however, was something of an eccentric, and his various foibles are well documented. He kept a pet hyena for a while, which he fed with live guinea pigs in order that he could study its poo in the context of a relatively 'natural' diet: indeed, he used his results to confirm hypotheses he had formulated on the basis of fossilised remains he had found in Kirkdale Cave, North Yorkshire. He was also an adventurous eater. He is, for example, said to have served mice on toast to his friends on more than one occasion (mice seem to have been a particular favourite of his; he also enjoyed them fried in batter) and to have eaten ostrich, rhino pie, panther chops, crocodile, bluebottle fly and mole (the latter two of which he pronounced the most disagreeable things he had ever eaten).

Buckland's son, Frank, inherited his father's eccentricities and took them a good deal further. His lifestyle led to the establishment of the bizarre (not to say barbaric) Victorian movement of 'zoophagy', literally the practice of dedicating oneself to eating one's way through the entire animal kingdom (his father also used to boast of this). Buckland is known to have eaten roast giraffe and elephant's trunk soup, and one year, on returning home from holiday, he learned that one of the leopards at London Zoo had died suddenly and had recently been buried in a flower bed. Buckland's reaction was to seize a spade, make his way to the zoo, dig up the leopard and eat it.

If all that wasn't macabre enough, Buckland's biographer (G. Burgess, *The Eccentric Ark: The Curious World of Frank Buckland*, 1967) reports that while he was training as a surgeon Buckland 'would often visit the local hospital in Winchester where he was on friendly terms with some of the staff and would exchange pieces of human anatomy for eels and trout'.

Jumble-giblets

Allow us for a moment to wear our backgrounds in linguistics on our sleeves. Consider the word 'giblets'. Firstly, while the word is always used in the plural, have you ever stopped to think what exactly it is the plural of? Just what is a 'giblet'? Is a heart, taken from a set of giblets (or, by extension, a gizzard, or a liver) a singular giblet? No. 'Giblets' shares with a small group of other words the property of being *plurale tantum*: the Latin for 'plural only'. Other examples include 'trousers', 'scissors' and 'clothes'.

And the etymology of 'giblets' is fascinating too, though tracing the history of words accurately is even more labyrinthine than cross-referencing fish species! The Merriam-Webster dictionary goes along with the claims of most etymologists, suggesting that the word's origins lie in the Frankish word *gibaiti*, which meant 'falconry'. From there it evolved via the Old French word *gibier*, 'game' or 'bird flesh', and *gibelet* – a ragout of game birds. Precisely when it came into English is unclear. Most sources suggest that it appeared around the thirteenth century and that its original meaning was, oddly enough, 'inessential appendages'. Within 100 years, however, it had come to mean what it does today. Ironically enough, given most people's attitude to giblets, the word it replaced was *garbage*, which, until the arrival of the word giblets (and the two words must have been synonymous for a while) then meant 'bird entrails'; in time, garbage evolved to mean 'waste' or 'refuse' in general. (In the US, garbage – or 'wet' waste, typically food – is still distinguished from trash, which is 'dry' waste.)

The etymological roots of the word gizzard, incidentally, lie in the Old French word *gisier*, which, you've guessed it, meant 'giblets'. And *gisier* evolved from the Latin term for 'giblets', *gigeria*, which itself came via the earlier Indo-European word *jigar*, meaning, er, 'liver'.

Confused? So are we.

The word *jigar* is still the word for 'liver' in Persian (and Hindi and Urdu), but the subtle processes responsible for language change have resulted in it having connotations that are unavailable to the English equivalent. When it is used figuratively, for example, *jigar* means 'courage' or 'conviction'. Indeed, in Urdu, *jan e jigar is* a term of endearment meaning, literally, 'strength of my liver'. This might explain why the title of the 1992 Bollywood revenge-blockbuster *Jigar* was translated into English as *Heart*.

While the term 'giblets' is generally used to describe a subset of the viscera found inside birds, differences in usage remain. The English version of *New Larousse Gastronomique* translates giblets into the French word *abatis*, which has a much broader meaning. On this broad construal, fowl giblets include the head, neck, heart, pinions (wing-tips), feet, liver, kidney, gizzard and, where appropriate, cocks' combs. In this volume we use the word in a slightly more restricted sense, to include the heart, gizzard and liver of any fowl. (Our restricted sense of the word is broader than the highly restricted sense defined in Allen and Gin, 1974. For them, the giblets are just the gizzard and the heart.) Continuing the etymological theme, perhaps unsurprisingly, the English word 'abattoir' is related to *abatis*, which evolved from the Old French *abattre*, meaning 'beaten down' or 'thrown down'. Less unsurprisingly, the English verb 'abate' also has its evolutionary roots in *abattre*, as does the now extinct verb 'bate', which lives on only in the phrase 'with bated breath'.

And in English the word 'giblets' has a slightly shady reputation thanks to its presence in some coarse slang phrases. According to the *Oxford English Dictionary,* in the 1800s and 1900s the verb phrase 'to join giblets' meant 'to marry'. From Jonathon Green's excellent *Dictionary of Slang*, however, we learn that the OFD may be guilty of exercising a little censorial licence: Green suggests that 'joining giblets' was actually used more often than not simply to refer to the action of having sexual intercourse, irrespective of whether the giblet joiners in question were married. The act has, at various times, also been variously referred to as 'rubbing offal' or 'giving someone some giblet pie' or (our favourite) 'performing the jumble-giblets'.

For many cultures, giblets – and livers in particular – have played a key cultural role. Ancient Greek soothsayers made prophecies solely on the basis of the condition of livers from sacrificed animals. Indeed, the Oracle of Delphi herself relied on close examination of animal livers to reassure herself that the time was right to prophesise. Hepatomancy, or as it came to be known, *haruspicy*, was central to the archaic religions of Ancient Rome, and so it was for the Etruscans too. As far as we know, it was the Ancient Babylonians who practised it first and they even had their own term for a person trained in the art: the *bãtû*. Many clay models of (in particular) sheeps livers survive to this day (there's one in the British Museum). The practice is even mentioned in the *Book of Ezekiel* 21:21.

> For the king of Babylon will stop at the fork in the road, at the junction of the two roads, to seek an omen: He will cast lots with arrows, he will consult his idols, he will examine the liver.

Heptomancy is less widespread nowadays, but does still exist. For the Daur ethnic group in China the wedding day of a couple is determined by examining the liver of a chick that the bride-and-groom-to-be have dispatched. If, as sometimes happens, the liver is for some reason not as it should be, the couple will be guided to another chick, which they will dissect in the hope of finding a more portentous liver. Quite what it is that makes one particular liver more reliable than any other when it comes to the organisation of nuptials we really have no idea. But chicken livers and joining giblets (or, more generally, giblet-jumbling) do at least enjoy a tenuous historical connection, and the idea that livers have qualities useful in divining the future is, as we have seen, not new.

Livers have other powers too. A tiny bit of duck liver is a popular homeopathic remedy for the flu. And when we say a tiny bit, we mean a really, really tiny bit: so tiny, in fact, that even the most ardent PETA activist need not worry. Perhaps conscious of the fact that not everyone likes the taste of duck liver, or perhaps wanting to keep as much of the liver as possible for their chicken liver pâté (recipe below), homeopaths recommend a 200C dilution. This is a solution of chicken liver that is so dilute that there be not a single molecule of liver in your prescription, or in a swimming pool – or (for that matter) a Pacific Ocean – filled with it. Indeed, if every subatomic particle in the known universe – every quark, gluon and recently-discovered Higgs boson – were expanded to the size of our universe and filled with the dilution, then in all those strange worlds, there would, perhaps, be just one lonely molecule of liver.

Even we had no idea quite how powerful the restorative properties of duck liver could be, and most of our friends think we're just a tad obsessed with the stuff.

This homeopathic remedy – *oscillococcinum* – also sometimes contains duck heart too (well, given the size of the known universe, it doesn't, but you know what we mean). But in general hearts seem not to have captured the imagination of soothsayers in the same way as livers. Regardless, various faiths ritually slaughter birds and make giblet offerings. Pity the pigeons and chickens (and water buffalo and pigs and goats) of the Bara District of

Nepal, some 150 kilometres south of Kathmandu. In the Gadhimai Festival of 2009, some 500,000 animals were sacrificed. Thankfully, the Chairman of the Gadhimai Temple, Mr Ram Chandra Shah, has decided that the next festival, in 2019, will involve no such bloodthirstiness.

As far as we know the Aztecs never saw sense in the same way: historian Fernando de Alva Cortés Ixtlilxóchitl, a direct descendant of an Aztec ruler, estimated one in five Aztec children were sacrificed to the gods. They were taken to the top of the local temple, eviscerated, and the priest would remove the still beating heart and offer it to the Gods in a ceremonial bowl.

And finally, from the truly macabre 'satansource' website comes the following suggestion as to how to best take revenge on a lover who has left you. Wait until midnight, take a bird's heart (many spiritualists favour swallow's heart, but we think chicken will probably do) and stick it full of pins. Safe in the knowledge that your ex-'s life is now completely ruined, prepare the garlic and lemon marinade we describe below and put the heart back in the fridge.

Revenge is best enjoyed char-grilled.

A bird's a bird

When buying birds, we adopt the same strategy as when buying fish: that is, we always try to buy the whole thing. The row upon row of brine-injected skinless chicken breast fillets in the supermarket is one of the worst example of that unhealthy disconnect between ingredient and source. If you want chicken, buy a chicken. One bird (and the same goes for all birds) will give a wide range of meals: take the breast fillets off, if you want, and poach them; remove the leg and roast them for another meal; after that you'll still have the meat on the carcass, and after that you'll still have the carcass itself, to make soup or stock. The whole bird is both more versatile and more economical (and let's try and get the giblets back).

Preparation and cooking

THE EASY WAY

The amount of work involved in the preparation of giblets depends entirely on the form in which you have bought them. If you have carefully sourced a ready-prepared bird with giblets, the likelihood is that they will already have been cleaned and will be residing in a small plastic bag within the cavity of the bird. If you have bought (or raised) a live bird, then there is more work to be done, not least in turning your live bird into one fit for the table.

There will be blood.

And how you buy your giblets will naturally dictate the recipe you choose. For physiological reasons we need hardly expand on, one chicken is not going

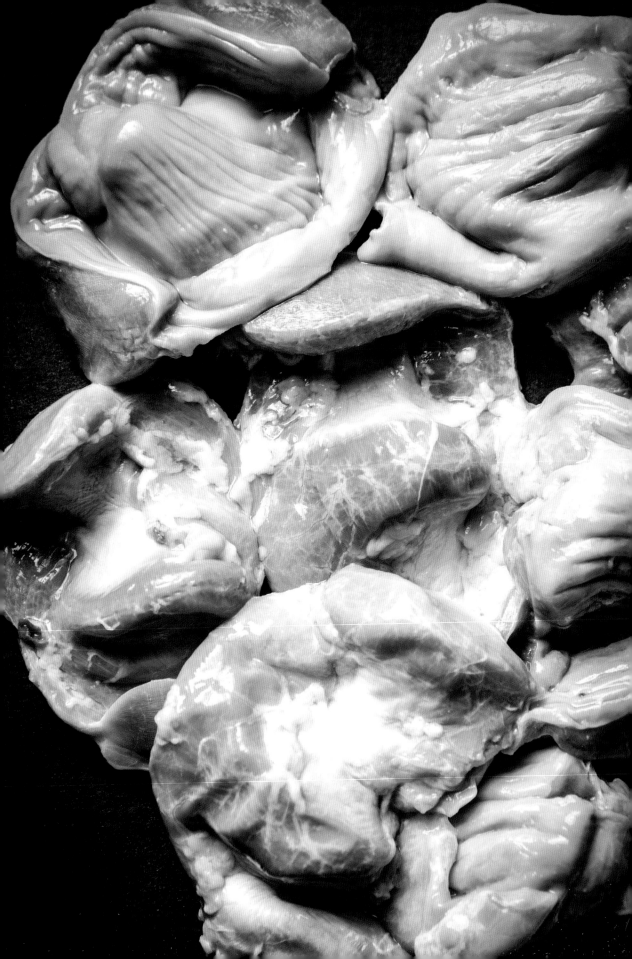

to supply you with enough hearts (nor gizzards, nor liver) to pack tightly on a metre long skewer and grill them *gaucho* style over charcoal. Still, many butchers will be able to sell you packs of pre-prepared hearts and gizzards, as well as tubs of livers. And it's a sad indictment on our cooking habits that you will always be able to find frozen hearts and gizzards in your local pet-shop. If you don't have a butcher nearby, check online. If we are going to encourage people to insist on the giblets coming with their bird, it seems to us that we have to get them to rediscover a taste for them first.

As far as cooking techniques are concerned, there is a range of different methods you can use. With the exception of the liver, all the other meats (so, the heart, gizzard, neck and wing-tips) work beautifully in slow cooked stews. As we say above, they add a real depth of flavour to just about any meat dish. However, liver simply doesn't work cooked in the same way: not only does it become as tough as leather, it's also likely to make your stock bitter. Far better to chop it (or them) finely, sauté in butter with garlic and enjoy on a crouton as a starter. As we say above, many people don't regard a bird's liver as part of the giblets at all: but it really is a part to cherish.

The only part of the giblets that doesn't respond well to quick cooking is the neck, which has to be cooked long and slow until what little meat is on it can be removed. Hearts and gizzards can both be cooked quite quickly (see the recipes). Leave your hearts whole, but chop the gizzards in two and, if anything, cook for slightly longer than the hearts.

Heart

Apart from taking care to remove all the voodoo pins (see above), there's very little you need to do to a fresh bird heart. Trim away any excess fat, although it is unlikely there will be much, and season liberally with salt and pepper and perhaps a pinch of mustard powder. Cook as per any of the delicious recipes that follow.

Liver

Make sure you check the livers for any green discolouring. If there is any, this is usually a sign that some bile has spilled on to the liver from the gall bladder: cut all the green away, since it may make the liver taste bitter. After that, we like soaking livers in milk before cooking them, particularly if it's that light creamy taste you're looking for – but if you're planning to grill them tandoori or yakitori style, or spice them up, we suggest you don't bother. Heart, liver and gizzard, we find, should be seasoned generously.

Gizzard

The gizzard is a bird's second stomach. Food passes from the crop first to the *proventriculus,* or 'true' stomach, where digestion begins, and is then transferred to the *ventriculus*, or gizzard ('gastric mill'), in which the food is properly broken down. Some species of birds, but not all, actively swallow stones (chickens do, and so do swallows), which help break food down when it is in the gizzard. The gizzard will probably already be cleaned and cut in half and, although larger, it will not be dissimilar in appearance to chicken hearts (sometimes hearts and gizzards are sold together in packs). If it's not cleaned, or if you've removed the gizzard yourself, you'll need to cut it in half, wash in a bowl of water to remove the grit that the bird uses to break food down, and cut away surrounding fat and the hard 'cap' at the top of the organ. You then need to cut away the wrinkled membrane and remove the dark morsels of meat inside. Even if they are pre-prepared, gizzards are slightly thicker and tougher than hearts and, as we say above, they consequently require slightly longer cooking. Some people advocate soaking gizzards for 15 minutes in vinegar, others overnight in milk or buttermilk. We ignore both strategies, unless we're making Southern Fried Gizzards (see page 237) and just slice them in two, lengthways (into conveniently heart-sized pieces), season them well and cook.

Neck

The neck that comes with your giblets will often come skinned. It's the bird's cervical vertebrae (and fused cervical ribs) which joins the backbone just behind the *furcula* (wishbone).

THE HARD(ER) WAY

If you've gone to the trouble of raising chickens or ducks, and you have a live one that you have singled out for the pot, then chances are you have already worked out how you're going to dispatch it. Besides, you've probably done it before. But if you have sourced a live bird, from a market say, then you will need to kill it. We have thought long and hard about how explicit to be in this regard. After all, we can hardly extol the virtues of being or becoming a smallholder and then provide instructions on the basics of butchering whilst ignoring the essential stage in between the two.

We gave our thoughts on this in the **Rabbits and Squirrels** chapter, and the same considerations apply to birds. So, if you have never slaughtered a chicken or duck before, we strongly advise you to get some guidance from

How to prepare fowl

Once the chicken or other fowl is dead, the procedure for preparation is as follows:

1. Scald the bird in a large pan of hot, but not boiling, water (60°C is fine). This will make plucking the bird easier.

2. Hang the bird upside down and carefully remove the feathers by pulling them downwards.

3. To clean the bird:

(a) Chop off the head.

(b) Slit the skin on the neck from the top of the backbone to the end of the neck.

(c) Separate the neck from the crop and the windpipe and throw away everything but the neck (which is great for stock).

(d) Cut a sharp incision at the back of the bird close to its cloaca. The cloaca is, in effect, a bird's anus, from where it passes urine and faeces. (It's also the orifice from where the hen lays eggs – one reason you should always wash your hands after handling eggs – and if you think that's a versatile orifice, some marine turtles actually breathe through their cloaca too).

(e) Put your hand inside the bird and remove all the innards.

(f) You are not really interested in the intestines, but you are interested in the heart, the gizzard and the liver.

(g) Remove the heart and trim off any fat.

(h) Take the gizzard, cut it in half lengthways and butterfly it open; it will probably contain the remains of the bird's last meal, and a few stones; remove any food that remains, and the stones, and rinse in cold water. Peel the ridged, yellow lining from the gizzard and rinse again.

(i) Take the liver, and remove the small bile duct; here's where you need to be careful not to spill any bile on the liver.

(j) Remove the chicken's feet; if you are going to eat these, you will need to scald them again and remove the 'socks' first.

Clean the inside of your chicken with a damp cloth and you are ready to go.

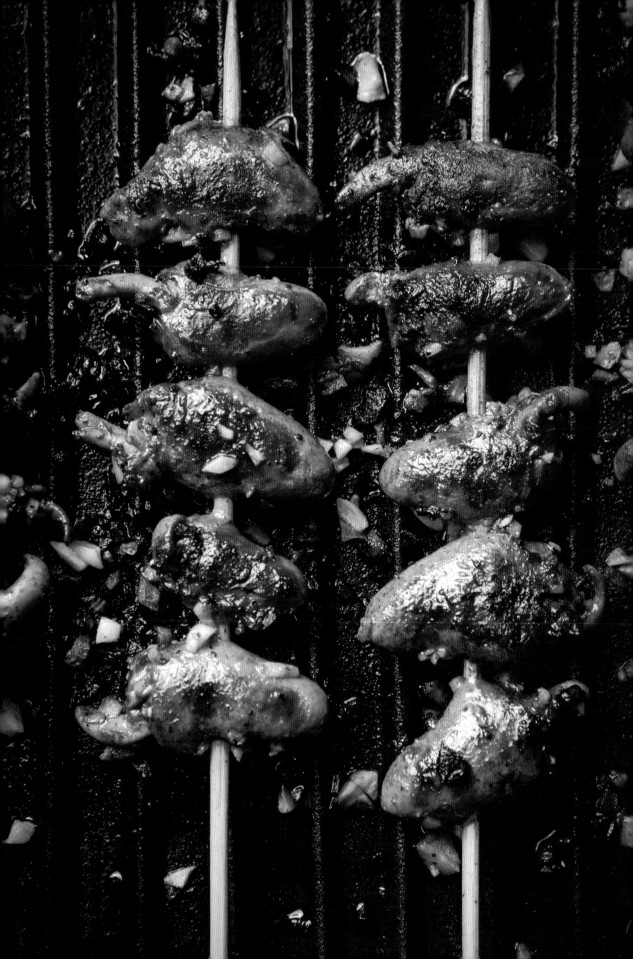

someone who has. Absolutely the last thing you want to do is cause the bird extra suffering. The most common slaughtering technique for home consumption is neck dislocation – a method whereby the neck is twisted quickly under the jaw, the spinal cord broken and blood flow to the brain arrested. This is permitted for birds weighing up to 3 kg (or up to 5 kg if a mechanical device is used). The two carotid arteries in the bird's neck must then be immediately cut, so that the bird bleeds out quickly and completely. Neck cutting should not be carried out without prior stunning. Commercial stunners are effective, and must be used on birds over 5 kg, but are expensive.

RECIPES

The gizzard of a domestic peacock and turkey cock are the most tasty of all birds' gizzards; if they are removed just as soon as the birds have been killed, they will be even tastier. If you want to roast them on a spit, more than half-cook them in salted water, then mount them on a slender spit, basting them with rendered fat and turning them slowly. Make up a mixture of flour, beaten egg yolks, sugar, saffron, rosewater and salt, giving it the consistency of a fritter batter; as the gizzards are cooking, baste on enough of that mixture that a crust is formed. Let them finish cooking until the batter is quite solid. Get very hot rendered fat with a spoon, brush it over them, then quickly sprinkle on fennel flour. Take them down and serve them hot with lime slices over them.

Bartolomeu Scappi, *Opera dell'Arte del Cucinare* (1570)

All recipes serve 4 unless otherwise noted.

Basic Giblet Soup

This is a basic soup recipe that can be augmented in a range of different ways to suit the style of soup you are looking for. With the addition of more meat (or just more giblets) you can turn it into a hearty stew. Many recipes call for the giblets of more than one bird: the supply problem can easily be overcome by either freezing giblets when you get them or, even better, preserving them in duck or goose fat (see our confit giblets recipe below).

500g assorted giblets (from chicken, duck, turkey or goose),
chopped into bite-size pieces
100g butter (or dripping or goose fat)
3 cloves of garlic, chopped
1 onion, chopped
1 leek, chopped

1 carrot, chopped

1 stick of celery, chopped

2 litres of stock

1 bay leaf

thyme

your preferred carbohydrate – this can be in the form of cooked rice, vermicelli or cubed potatoes

salt and freshly-ground black pepper

1. Melt the fat in a large saucepan.

2. Brown the assorted giblets. Remove when nicely browned and reserve.

3. Add the garlic and vegetables to the fat in the pan and brown a little.

4. Add the stock, bay leaf and thyme. Bring to the boil and then reduce the heat so that the soup plops or bubbles rather than trots or gallops. You want to keep it simmering very gently for an hour or so, or until everything is nicely cooked through; if potato is your carbohydrate of choice, add cubed pieces about 20 minutes from the end of the cooking time. If you're adding vermicelli, add it to the soup 2 minutes before eating; if you're adding cooked rice, add it about a minute before. Serve.

The original recipe on which this is based – one from Alexis Soyer's *A Shilling Cookery for the People* – is based on a roux of flour and fat. We prefer the looser, more brothy version above. If you like a slightly thicker sauce (as indeed Escoffier does in his recipe for *Soupe aux Abatis de Volaille a l'Anglaise*) add a tablespoonful of plain flour to the giblets in the pan at stage 2, leave them in your pan while you brown your garlic and vegetables and then add the stock as instructed.

And while it is a simple soup, it can be used as the basis for a whole range of hearty dishes. A few options follow:

- Cook some haricot beans with a small piece of salt pork or bacon (I use the end piece of Parma ham that my local delicatessen owner sells me once he can no longer slice from it), then proceed as above and add beans and bacon together with the stock in stage 4. Fergus Henderson gives a beautiful recipe along these lines for the St. John 'giblet stew' in his book *Nose to Tail Eating* – he uses confit giblets, for which see the recipe below.

- Add some of the meat from the bird whose giblets you have used (or more giblets – see the goose giblet version below).

- Add any white meat, but make sure it is suited to long slow cooking (see Cheeks and Feet chapter): belly pork would be perfect, tenderloin a disaster.

- In *Innards and Other Variety Meats*, Allen and Gin provide a recipe for 'German giblet soup' which uses chicken wings as well as the giblets, and is finished with some double cream: this is delicious too.

As with all the options we suggest to augment our recipes throughout the book, keep the MAXIM OF PURITY in mind.

Confit Giblets

If you are fortunate to find a source of fresh duck or goose giblets, grab the lot. Confit is the perfect way to both cook and store them. The basic idea is simple. Meat that is covered in fat is, effectively, in an air-free environment. The bacteria that spoil meats can't survive without air, so the meat will last for ages. It's true that nowadays most people's favoured method of food preservation is freezing, but this often reduces the quality of the finished product. If anything, confiting improves it!

Giblets (duck or goose are best) – gizzards, hearts, necks (eat the liver fresh)

enough duck or goose fat to cover the giblets (you can buy goose fat in many supermarkets these days, but if you have roast goose at Christmas, you will be amazed how much fat it will give you)

salt and freshly-ground black pepper

twigs of thyme

1. In a non-metallic container strew coarse salt, pepper and twigs of thyme.

2. Place some giblets on the top in one layer.

3. Cover the giblets with salt, pepper and thyme and repeat to give as many layers as you need to use up all the giblets.

4. Cover the container and place in the fridge for 24 hours.

5. Throw away the liquid that will have emerged during this time and brush off all the salt that remains on the giblets; wipe them with a cloth or tea towel.

6. Place the giblets in an oven dish, cover with fat and cook in a 190°C oven for about 2 hours. The giblets will be well cooked but you want to keep them the solid side of falling apart.

7. Once cooked, remove the giblets and reserve. Separate any meat juices from the fat, which is essential if you want to keep the confit more than a couple of weeks – you don't need to worry about this step if you plan to eat them within that time. For easy removal of the meat juices, we find putting the fat in the fridge until the two have separated and the fat has solidified works well. Don't throw these juices out – they are liquid gold for stocks or adding to sauces.

8. Place the giblets in a non-metallic container once more; ideally, you want a china crock with a top that narrows in order that you need less fat to keep it all well and truly covered. Cover with the fat and make sure there are no giblets poking through.

9. Store for up to six months (we don't go longer than that, but you probably could).

All you need to do to prepare your giblets for eating is heat them in the fat in which they been preserved. Chop them finely and serve them in a salad with mustard-heavy vinaigrette, such as the one in the recipe for Head Salad on page 72. Alternatively, use them in the basic giblet soup above.

Don't throw the fat away. Simply strain it and use for your next batch of confit.

Mizutaki

Here is another Fukuoka recipe from Akiko Tsuda and Norio Matsukuma. Fukuoka is a town on the northern-most tip of Kyushu, and *mizutaki* is a dish that is now renowned all over the country. There are two versions, one featuring a broth that is made milky by the addition of ground chicken bones, the other with a clear, consommé-like soup. This recipe is for the former version.

The original recipe calls for a whole chicken portioned into 50g pieces. This is not that difficult if you know what you're doing, but since it's an unfamiliar way of portioning a chicken, it can be quite challenging for a home cook. In the following recipe, we've suggested removing the legs, wings and the breast fillets from the chicken and then chopping the remaining carcass into small pieces to make a stock. You can then cut the breast pieces and the legs into small pieces (chopping the legs with a cleaver or sharp knife is easy). If you're confident you can portion the chicken into 50g pieces, go ahead.

A note on the Japanese ingredients: Most of these ingredients are easily available in Japanese groceries, or even many Western supermarkets, including chrysanthemum leaves (which have a distinct flavour that goes very well with chicken), *konegi* (a vegetable that is half way between a spring onion and a leek – if you can't get it, use the green part of a spring onion), Ponzu sauce (a popular Japanese citrus-soy sauce mixture) and *Momiji oroshi* (you can buy this in tubes like wasabi, but you can also easily make your own, and it's much better – finely grate some daikon, mix with a little finely chopped dried red chilli, then put in a small piece of cheesecloth and squeeze out any excess moisture; serve immediately).

1 chicken with giblets

2 litres water

4 shitake mushrooms, quartered

a quarter of a Chinese cabbage, chopped

150g cauliflower

20g sliced *konegi* leek

1 block firm tofu, cut into squares

Ponzu sauce

Momiji oroshi (grated daikon radish with red chilli)

a bunch of chrysanthemum leaves (*shungiku* or *kikuna* in Japanese)

1. Prepare the chicken. First, chop the giblets (do not use the liver) and set aside. Next, remove the legs, wings and breast fillets from the chicken and put aside. Then chop the remaining carcass into small pieces.

2. Rinse your chopped chicken carcass and place it in a pot with the water and a little salt; simmer for about half an hour. Remove some of the bones and grind them in a mortar; return to the stock, which should now go milky.

3. Cut the legs, wings and breast into pieces. Place the leg and wing pieces in a deep pot and add the milky stock; bring to a rolling simmer and cook for 15 minutes, being careful to remove any scum that comes to the surface; add the pieces of breast and the chopped giblets and cook for 10 minutes more.

4. Add the vegetables and tofu to the stock; place the Ponzu and *Momiji oroshi* in small bowls.

Mizutaki is a 'hotpot' dish so traditionally it would be presented on a table-top burner or hotplate, so that it will continue to cook slowly as you eat. The idea is that you help yourself to the tofu, various vegetables and chicken and eat them with the two accompaniments. When only the stock is left, cook some udon noodles in it and serve them, with the remaining stock, in individual bowls.

Braised Gizzards with Black Bean Sauce

500g gizzards

generous splash of soy sauce

generous splash of Chinese cooking wine (or dry sherry)

30g root ginger, finely sliced

2 cloves of garlic, finely chopped

50g fermented black beans, mashed

pinch of sugar

neutral vegetable oil

500ml chicken stock

a tablespoon of cornflour mixed with double the quantity of cold water

1. Cut the gizzards into two pieces along the centre.

2. Mix together the soy, wine, ginger, garlic, black beans and sugar. Add the gizzards to the mixture and marinate for one hour.

3. Heat some vegetable oil in a saucepan or wok and add the gizzards; fry them until lightly browned.

4. Add the stock, bring to the boil and then simmer for between 45 minutes and 1 hour.

5. Before serving thicken with the cornflour and water mixture. Test the seasoning, adding more soy if necessary; a light sprinkle of sesame oil is also nice.

6. Serve with steamed rice.

Crisp Fried Hearts and Gizzards

500g prepared hearts and gizzards

about 120g flour

about 30g cornflour

oil for frying

For the marinade:

healthy splash of soy sauce

an equally healthy splash of Chinese rice wine or dry sherry

30g root ginger, grated

2 cloves of garlic, grated or finely chopped

3 spring onions, very finely sliced

1 bird's-eye chilli, very finely sliced

1. Assemble the marinade and add the hearts and gizzards, leaving for an hour or two.

2. Add the flour and the cornflour to the hearts, the gizzards and the marinade.

3. Mix together briefly – you are aiming at a consistency where the now floury marinade is clinging (albeit in an irregular, slightly lumpy way) to the meat.

4. Heat the oil in your deep-fryer to 180°C and fry the hearts and gizzards for between 3–5 minutes.

5. The end product should be dark brown and nicely crisp. Serve with more soy and Thai sweet chilli sauce.

Southern Fried Gizzards

In many of the southern states of the US, KFC include a liver and/or gizzard meal on their menu (with mashed potato, gravy and flaky buttermilk biscuit). Pressure cooking before frying is the best way to get tender gizzards; if you don't have a pressure cooker, an alternative is to soak the gizzards in buttermilk for 24 hours.

500g of gizzards

flour

seasoning mix (see below)

For years, the secret blend of eleven herbs and spices in KFC seasoning was a closely guarded trade secret. Here's how to make it:

1 teaspoon each of: oregano, chilli powder, dried sage, dried basil, dried marjoram, onion salt, garlic powder, black pepper

2 teaspoon each of: salt, paprika (not the smoked variety), Accent™ – an MSG-based seasoning powder available in online food stores
(it contains colours too)

Experiment with the ratio of the seasoning to flour; as a general rule of thumb you want enough seasoning mix for the flour to be nicely coloured.

1. Cut the gizzards into bite-size pieces. Place in a pressure cooker with enough water or chicken stock to barely cover and cook at full pressure for 20 minutes. Once the cooker has depressurised, remove the gizzards, drain and allow to cool, then pat dry.

2. Coat the gizzards in the seasoned flour mix.

3. Heat the oil in a deep fat fryer to 180°C; fry the gizzards for 3 minutes, until they are crisp and golden.

Darn tootin'.

MSG is not evil

We don't have a problem with monosodium glutamate. It's a naturally-occurring substance used all around the world as a flavour enhancer – providing a hit of savoury umami, the so-called 'sixth taste'. And while we don't advocate adding it to everything as a substitute for cooking decent flavourful food, it definitely has its place in seasonings, mayonnaise and so on. If you want to avoid it, you can always add more salt....

Corações de Galinhas Grelhado

Porto Alegre is a city of about 1.5 million inhabitants in the far south of Brazil. It's gaucho country and the locals are fiercely proud of their culinary heritage. Just as the gauchos roast their meat over an open fire on huge, metre-long skewers, so the local churrascarias serve an array of grilled meats that have been cooked over charcoal: among the variety of meats available there will be many different types of beef – sirloin steak, rump steak (and top-rump or *picanha*), feather steak (with and without garlic) and beef rib; pork – ribs, smoked leg, leg with garlic and spices, spicy pork sausages and ham with pineapple; chicken – spicy chicken legs and chicken with; lamb – leg steaks, slow roast shoulder and lamb cutlets.

But the highlight, to our minds, was these simply mind-blowingly delicious skewers of chicken hearts, first marinated in lime and garlic. *São maravilhosos*!

as many hearts as you can lay your hands on
juice of several limes
half a dozen cloves of garlic
salt, pepper and mustard powder

1. Squeeze the juice from the limes into a bowl. Grate or finely chop the garlic and add to the lime. Add the chicken hearts.

2. If you have a charcoal grill, all the better, but we find cast-iron ridged grill pans to be an excellent substitute. Simply heat the pan. Thread the hearts onto a skewer or skewers, season well with salt, pepper and mustard powder (or cayenne pepper) and grill.

Eat piping hot with a beer or, even better, a caipirinha.

You can adapt this recipe by adding spices to the garlic marinade; the marinade in the following recipe would work perfectly.

Tandoori Chicken Livers

Nearly everyone knows that the *tandoori* part of the name of any Indian dish refers to the clay oven – the tandoor – in which it is cooked. In English, however, the word is used to refer to the spice-mixture in which the meat or fish is marinated before cooking. You might be surprised to learn that as linguists, we have no prescriptive point to make about this; as far as we're concerned, what words mean is a matter of what people mean by them.

Pre-prepared 'tandoori' marinades are available in supermarkets and Indian stores but we find they vary in quality hugely and encourage you to try making your own. These livers are undoubtedly better char-grilled, but they take so little time, you might feel that lighting and tending a fire is a little too much trouble. Our solution is to marinate chicken thighs, hearts ('chicken ticker'?) and gizzards too and have ourselves a Punjabi feast! If you want to do this, follow the recipe below, making double the amount of marinade, and adding 500g of chicken thighs and some hearts.

500g chicken livers

For the marinade (double the quantities if you are making our Punjabi feast):

15g root ginger, grated
2 cloves of garlic, grated or finely chopped

100g natural yoghurt

equal quantities of: ground turmeric, ground cumin, ground cinnamon, chilli powder (as much as you like – we like a lot), black pepper, garam masala; we try to avoid using 'teaspoon' as a volume measure but it works with spices, so half a teaspoon of each is fine

juice of half a lemon

salt (plenty)

1. Make the marinade by mixing together all the ingredients. Add the chicken livers to half the marinade and marinate for at least twelve hours.

2. Thread the livers on to short metal or wooden skewers (pre-soaked in water to prevent them burning).

3. Grill over charcoal, or on a cast-iron ridged grill pan (as per the chicken hearts above).

4. Serve with chopped fresh coriander and flatbreads.

Chicken Heart and Gizzard Yakitori

The traditional Japanese yakitori marinade makes a valuable addition to your repertoire.

500g chicken hearts and gizzards

spring onions

For the marinade:

60ml soy sauce

60ml mirin

15g sugar

2 cloves garlic, finely chopped

1. Wash the hearts and gizzards thoroughly; slice them into bite-size pieces (this is important, if the pieces are too big, the yakitori will be difficult to eat).

2. Put the marinade ingredients in a small pan; bring to the boil and simmer until the liquid thickens (3–5 minutes).

3. Pour half the marinade over the hearts and gizzards, saving the other half for later; place the hearts and gizzards in the fridge and leave for a minimum of 3 hours.

4. Once the meat is in the fridge, soak some bamboo skewers in water.

5. Thread the hearts and gizzards on to the bamboo skewers and grill them on your cast-iron ridged griddle pan. Be careful, though; you do not want the pan to be quite as hot as it is in the previous recipe, as the marinade has a tendency to burn, so be gentle. (A charcoal grill is the traditional way of cooking yakitori.)

6. Present the yakitori on a bed of chopped spring onion and brush with the remaining marinade.

Chicken Liver and Sage Bruschetta

This is a delicious starter or, served with a green salad, makes a lovely light lunch. Many recipes call for livers to be cooked slowly in butter, but we prefer olive oil and a hot pan. (You can then add a little butter once they are cooked.) Experiment and see which method you prefer.

250g chicken liver

some milk

olive oil

2 cloves of garlic, finely chopped

4 large sage leaves, roughly chopped

a small knob of butter

plenty of salt and pepper

slices of toasted bread (bruschetta)

1. Remove and discard any green bits from the liver (the colour comes from bile released by the gall bladder and it can make the liver taste bitter). Soak the liver in milk for an hour or so and then drain and pat dry.

2. Chop the livers into a smallish dice.

3. Heat a tablespoon of olive oil in a large frying pan until hot and then add the livers in one go. There will be a lot of sizzling and spitting, but take courage and leave the livers alone for ten seconds or so – do not be tempted to move them around.

4. Once the sizzling and spitting subsides, add the garlic, sage and butter and move the livers around the pan for another ten seconds or so; you are aiming for a little char on the outside and pinkness on the inside.

5. Season well. (At this stage, you can purée the liver mixture in a blender if you like, but we prefer not to.)

6. Pile the liver, garlic and sage mixture on the bruschetta. Serve, accompanied by dry white wine.

Devilled Chicken Livers

This recipe is from Sir Harry Luke's delightful book *The Tenth Muse*, attributed to one Mrs John Stone of Malta.

6 chicken livers

20ml Worcestershire sauce

20ml tomato sauce (we use ketchup)

1 tablespoon Madras curry powder

40g butter

Warm the butter in a pan, add the Worcestershire and tomato sauces with the curry powder. Simmer and cook for a quarter of an hour, chop the livers very fine and add to the mixture, cooking slowly for another 15 minutes. Serve on toast, very hot. This should be cooked at the last moment...

Try it. You won't be disappointed.

Gänsekleinsuppe

Goose giblet soup with dumplings. The addition of dried fruit is typical of the cooking of Schleswig-Holstein.

1kg goose or duck giblets (and wings too)

1.5 litres water

2 bay leaves

4 whole cloves

goose or duck fat

1 onion, finely chopped

1 carrot, finely chopped

1 stick of celery, finely chopped

75g of dried apple slices, chopped

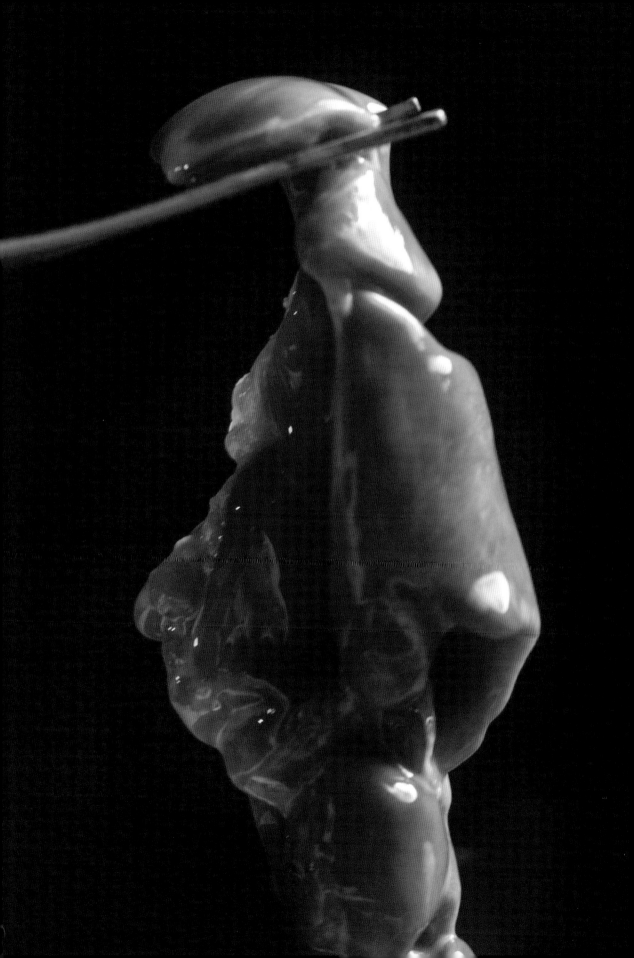

75g of dried apricot, chopped

10 prunes, chopped

50ml of cider vinegar

enough sugar to give the final dish a sweet-sour taste

salt and freshly-ground black pepper

For the dumplings:

1kg red potatoes

1 egg, lightly beaten

50g duck fat, melted

50g breadcrumbs

125g plain flour

salt and freshly-ground black pepper

1. Pre-heat the oven to 200°C.

2. Remove the liver from the giblets, it will make the soup bitter if included (you can keep it for one of the liver recipes in this chapter, or chopped, lightly sautéed and served alongside the soup). Place the rest of the giblets in a large pot and cover with water; add the bay leaves, cloves and a little salt; bring to the boil, remove any scum that rises to the surface, cover and cook in the oven for about 3 hours, or until the meat is beginning to fall off the wings.

3. Meanwhile, you can start making the dumpling dough. Place your potatoes in the oven too and bake them for about an hour until they are good and soft.

4. While the potatoes are cooking, caramelise the onion slowly in a pan with some goose or duck fat; it's fine if it browns a little (in fact, that's what you're looking for), but don't let it burn. Once the onion is nicely coloured and softened, add the carrot, celery and fruit and cook for another 5–10 minutes.

5. When the potatoes are cooked, put them through a potato ricer. All you need to do is cut the potatoes in half around the equator and the potato will emerge, beautifully riced, leaving the skins in the ricer. (If you don't have a potato ricer, remove the skins and mash; but you should get a ricer – they make absolutely the best mashed potato in the world.)

6. Put the potato in a mixing bowl. Add the egg, fat, breadcrumbs, flour, salt and pepper and mix them until you have dough that is still a little sticky, but just holds together. You need to be gentle. Don't work the dough the way you might bread dough, if you do, the dumplings will be unpleasant and heavy.

7. Once the meat is tender, remove the pan from the oven and take out the giblets and wings. Roughly chop the giblets and pull off the meat from the neck and wings. Return all of the meat to the soup. Add the browned onion, celery, carrot, and dried fruit. Add the sugar and vinegar to taste and make sure you have that nice sweet-sour piquancy. Turn on the heat again and bring the soup back to a simmer.

8. Take small handfuls of the dumpling mixture and form them into balls about the size of a small plum. Drop them into the soup. After 4–5 minutes they should come to the surface; this means they are done – remove the cooked dumplings and reserve.

9. Serve the soup hot in deep bowls; top with dumplings.

Chicken Liver Pâté (Pâté de Foie)

This pâté is very rich and we find that a little goes a long way. This makes enough for 4 people as a starter, or as part of a light lunch.

200g chicken livers

200g unsalted butter (room temperature)

1 clove of garlic, very finely chopped

1 shallot, very finely chopped

30ml brandy

dash of Dijon mustard

ground allspice

salt and freshly-ground black pepper

1. Clarify 100g of the butter – simply heat it gently, skimming off any solids that rise to the surface; when all the solids are gone from the top, let the butter settle for 2 minutes and pour off the golden clarified butter (through muslin – or an old tea-strainer) leaving the remaining solids at the bottom of the pan. Reserve the clarified butter for use in stage 8.

2. Add 50g butter to a frying pan and gently cook the garlic and shallot.

3. Add the chicken livers and cook them very slowly (you don't want them to colour) for around 5 minutes; you should turn them once; prod them with your finger – they should never get beyond the point where they are soft and yielding.

4. Take the chicken livers out of the pan, put them in a bowl and add the brandy to the pan; turn the heat up a little and make sure all the juices in the pan mix with the brandy.

5. Add the brandy to the livers and the final 50g of butter; add a dash of mustard, a grating of allspice, a large pinch of salt and a good couple of twists of pepper.

6. Put everything in a blender and blend very well.

7. Sieve the mixture into a white serving dish (or individual ones are nice).

8. Seal your pâté(s) with the clarified butter.

9. Cover with foil or cling-film, place in the fridge and wait for a couple of days before serving. Eat with bread or toast and some gherkins or other pickles.

You can, if you like, replace the butter added at stage 5 with double cream. Also, while we like this with brandy, and the dish does need that background kick, you could try another alcohol. We have found many recipes calling for Madeira and others that use port (the recipe below uses Marsala). Experiment and discover which you like best. This recipe is also nice with duck or goose livers, if you can get them, as is the following recipe.

Chicken Liver Sauce for Pasta

500g chicken liver, cut into small pieces

50g unsalted butter

1 shallot, finely chopped

15g tomato purée

50ml Marsala (you can use dry white wine instead,
but Marsala will give you a better flavour)

30g dried porcini mushrooms, soaked in hot water and chopped

1. Melt the butter in a pan and cook the shallot gently for 5–10 minutes.

2. Add the chicken livers and cook them gently for another 5 minutes or so.

3. Stir in the tomato purée, Marsala and porcini.

4. Stir well, reducing the Marsala a little, and thin to a sauce-like consistency with the water in which the porcini have been soaked (being careful to leave any grit behind – or you can strain it first through a coffee filter or muslin).

5. Serve with tagliolini and shavings of white truffle.

You probably won't have white truffles, but the suggestion that you add them is no mere luxurious whim. This sauce is from Piedmont in northern Italy, the centre of the white truffle trade, and the combination of white truffles with the sauce (and *tajarin*, the local name for tagliolini) is wonderful.

The sauce is also excellent stirred into a plain risotto or, for that matter, just-cooked long-grain rice. It's also excellent with polenta.

Pollo Orvietano (Orvieto Chicken)

This is a perfect example of how the giblets can contribute so much more to a chicken dish than just flavouring the gravy. Alastair Little calls this recipe 'ravishing' and who are we to disagree with him?

1 free-range chicken with giblets – 1.5-2kg

1 onion, diced

50ml extra virgin olive oil

3 heads of garlic
(separated into cloves – two cloves peeled and finely chopped)

500g potatoes, cut into 1cm dice

1 bulb fennel, diced

1 lemon

200g black olives
(don't buy pitted olives, just crush olives on your board
and the stone will come out easily)

sprigs of rosemary and thyme

150 ml of dry white wine (Orvieto would be perfect)

salt and freshly-ground black pepper

1. Sauté the diced onion and chopped giblets in about half the olive oil (but don't allow the onion to brown); add the two chopped cloves of garlic, the potato and fennel and continue to sauté for 10–15 minutes until the vegetables are nicely cooked; allow to cool slightly.

2. Season the vegetable and giblet mix well, add some lemon juice and then stuff it into the cavity of the chicken; use a couple of skewers to keep the cavity closed.

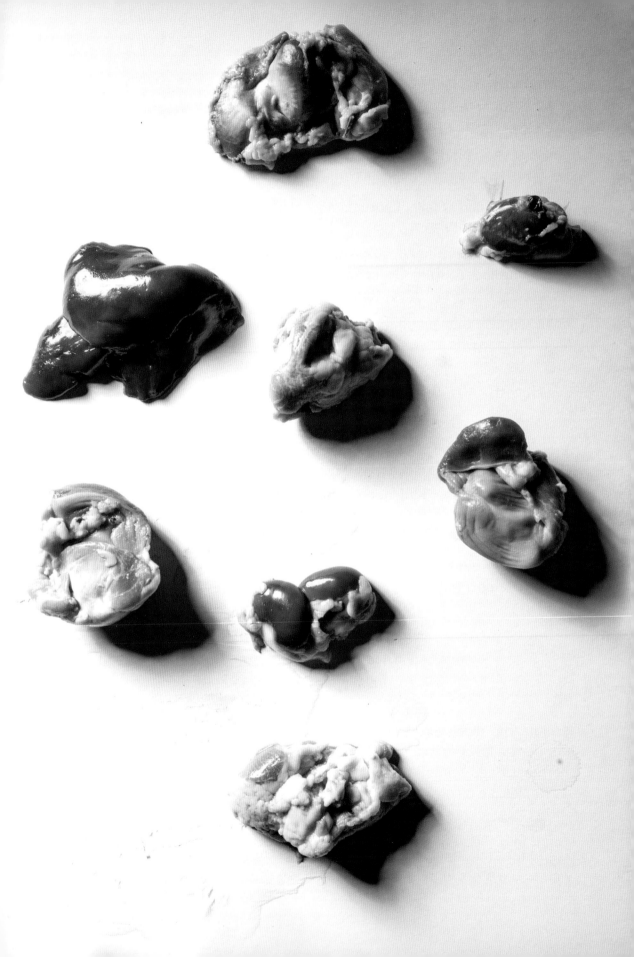

There are many different ways to roast a chicken. We prefer Thomas Keller's straightforward method, described below: no moving, no basting.

3. Season the skin of the bird all over with salt and pepper and place on its back in an oven pre-heated to 200°C.

4. After around 40 minutes, remove the chicken from the oven and strew the olives, herbs and unpeeled garlic cloves all around it; also add a little water and the rest of the olive oil (just into the dish – don't baste the bird itself).

5. Once it's cooked (if you have a probe thermometer, you're looking for something like an internal temperature of 65°C in the thickest part of the leg), remove the bird from the pan and leave to rest in a warm place for at least 15 minutes (preferably half an hour).

6. Pour the excess fat out of the roasting pan then deglaze the pan with the white wine; this will give you a thin, but sumptuous gravy.

7. Remove the stuffing from the inside of the bird and place it on a large serving platter; portion the bird into 8 pieces (each leg and each breast into 2).

Hungarian Sauté of Hearts and Gizzards

1kg hearts and gizzards

flour

50g butter or duck fat (or chicken fat)

1 tablespoon smoked paprika (not the spicy variety)

125ml white wine

125ml chicken stock

2 cloves of garlic, finely chopped

1 red onion, finely sliced

1 red pepper, finely sliced

fresh thyme

salt and freshly-ground black pepper

250ml sour cream

1. Dust the hearts and gizzards in a generous quantity of flour and brown them well in the butter or oil; add the paprika and mix well on the heat.

2. Add the wine, bring to a simmer, flame off the alcohol, then add the stock with all the other ingredients apart from the sour cream.

3. Cover and simmer for about an hour.

4. Reduce the sauce to a thick consistency, season well with salt and pepper, and then add the sour cream.

5. Serve with noodles.

Giblet Pie

Let's face it. When all is said and done, sometimes we all fancy a little slice of giblet pie. This is the recipe Escoffier provides in his *Guide to the Art of Modern Cookery* (1903). You'll need about 500g of giblets, and, if you don't make your own puff pastry (and we don't), buy 500g of the ready-rolled variety. Use stock (giblet stock if you have some frozen) instead of consommé.

Fry the giblets, cut into pieces, in butter; sprinkle them moderately with flour; cook the latter, and moisten with just sufficient consommé to make a clear sauce which will just cover the pieces. Three-parts cook, and leave to cool.

This done, pour the whole into a pie-dish; cover with a layer of puff-paste, which should be sealed down to a strip of paste, stuck to the edge of the dish; gild; streak, and bake in a moderately warm oven for from 25–30 minutes.

To modern cooks, the terms 'gild' and 'streak' are unfamiliar in the context of recipes. By 'gild' Escoffier means apply egg-wash. To 'streak' pastry ('paste') is to break its surface lightly with the prongs of a fork in order to increase the surface area exposed to the heat. We both gild, but only one of us streaks (and very occasionally at that).

Alicot d'Oie aux Legumes d'Hiver
(Goose Giblets with Root Vegetables)

This recipe is from Pierre Koffman's delightful book *Memories of Gascony*. We have to confess that we've never made it with just goose giblets. While the goose plays a huge role in Gascon peasant life and cookery, it is quite a luxury in the UK, where a good size bird (which won't give you enough giblets for this recipe) will cost you around £70 – and only feed six at a stretch. If you keep geese (and we salute you if you do), this is a recipe for you. Also, where do you live? If you can't get goose giblets, the recipe is just as delicious made with duck giblets.

1–1.5kg goose giblets: including necks, wings, gizzards, livers, hearts, feet (or the same weight of duck giblets)

80g goose or duck fat

200g bacon, diced into lardons

300g onion, chopped

300ml dry white wine

bunch of thyme and a couple of bay leaves

6 garlic cloves, crushed

100g each of chopped leeks, carrots, potatoes, turnips and pumpkin

half a savoy cabbage, diced

1. Heat the goose/duck fat in a deep, heavy casserole and fry the bacon quite hard until coloured; remove the bacon and add the giblets (apart from the liver); let them brown too, add the onion, reduce the heat and cook for 10 more minutes or so until the onion has softened.

2. Pour in the wine, add enough water to make sure the giblets are covered, and then add the bacon back to the pan with the herbs and garlic; season well and bring back to a gentle simmer.

3. After 45 minutes add the leeks and carrots and continue simmering; after 5 more minutes add the potato; and after another 10 minutes add the turnip, cabbage and pumpkin.

4. A further 15 minutes later, so after about an hour and a quarter cooking, everything should be good and tender.

5. Pan fry the livers in fat until they are nice and pink in the middle; add them to the stew.

6. Before serving, check for seasoning.

Celeriac or mangel-wurzel would be happy substitutes for turnips in this recipe.

Alycuit à l'occitane is a related dish from Languedoc, the region to the east of Gascony, in which the root vegetables above are replaced with tomatoes, artichoke hearts and peas. This gives the dish a wonderfully summery lightness (in Autumn, the Languedoc tradition is to add wild mushrooms and chestnuts – we've found dried porcini and pre-cooked chestnuts work really nicely). For the summer version add the tomatoes and artichokes at stage 3 instead of the root vegetables and add the peas about 10 minutes before the dish is ready.

Peas, of course, will be familiar to all readers. However, while grown and devoured in their millions in continental Europe, globe artichokes are rarely seen in the UK, either in our fields, in our shops or on our tables: this despite the fact that they grow perfectly well here and are delicious. Precisely why it is that UK consumers eschew the albeit rather unprepossessing set of flower heads that grow from the central, also edible, bud (known as the 'heart') of *cynara scolymus* – essentially a thistle – we have no idea.

And this seems neither the time nor the place to discuss why.

INDEX

Entries in **bold** indicate recipes

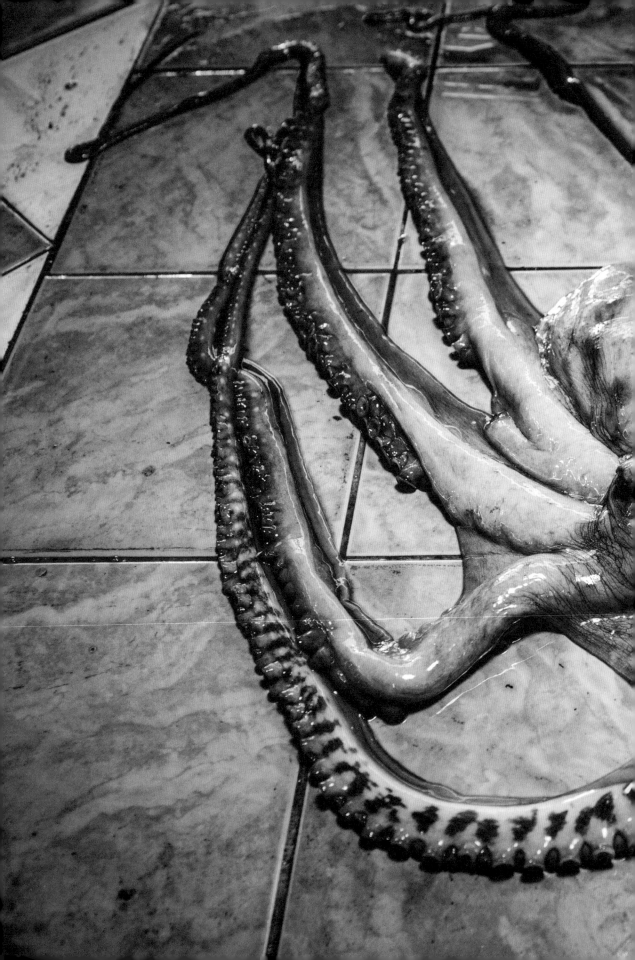

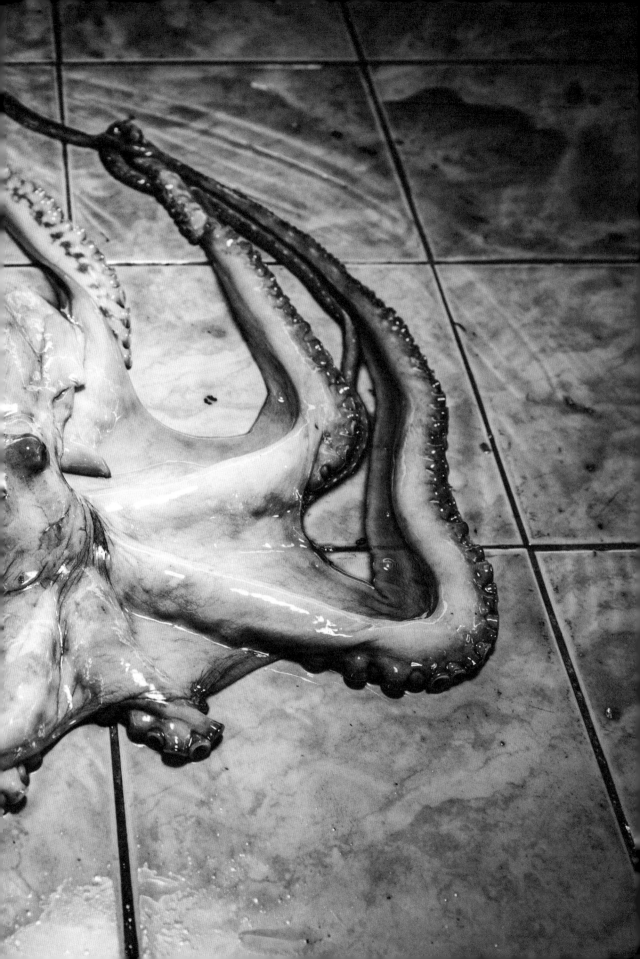

31192021389620